new-style
Tai Chi Ch'uan

The Official Chinese System

Wei Yue Sun, M.D.
& Xiao Jing Li, M.D.

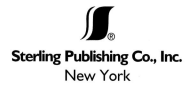

Sterling Publishing Co., Inc.
New York

Photography by Sung Kwan Ma
Edited with page layouts by Jeanette Green

Library of Congress Cataloging-in-Publication Data

Sun, Wei Yue.
    New style Tai chi ch'uan : the official Chinese system / Wei Yue
Sun, Xiao Jing Li.
        p.   cm.
    Includes index.
    ISBN 0–8069–9703–6
    1. Tai chi ch'uan.   I. Li, Xiao Jing.   II. Title.   III. Title:
Tai chi ch'uan.
GV504.S85   1999
613.7' 148–dc21   99–21090

10 9 8 7 6 5 4 3 2 1
Published by Sterling Publishing Company, Inc.
387 Park Avenue South, New York, N.Y. 10016
© 1999 by Wei Yue Sun and Xiao Jing Li
Distributed in Canada by Sterling Publishing
c/o Canadian Manda Group, One Atlantic Avenue, Suite 105
Toronto, Ontario, Canada M6K 3E7
Distributed in Great Britain and Europe by Cassell PLC
Wellington House, 125 Strand, London WC2R 0BB, England
Distributed in Australia by Capricorn Link (Australia) Pty Ltd.
P.O. Box 6651, Baulkham Hills, Business Centre, NSW 2153, Australia
Manufactured in the United States of America

Sterling ISBN 0—8069—9703—6

Contents

UNDERSTANDING TAI CHI CH'UAN   5

The History of Tai Chi Ch'uan   7

The Philosophy of Tai Chi Ch'uan—*Yin & Yang*   12

The Physiology of Tai Chi Ch'uan—*The Channels & Meridians*   15

Meditation—*The Flow of Chi through Channels & Meridians*   21

Breathing—*The Exercise of Yin & Yang*   23

The Physical Movements of Tai Chi Ch'uan   25

The Health Benefits of Tai Chi Ch'uan   27

Tai Chi Ch'uan & Self-Defense   30

NEW-STYLE TAI CHI CH'UAN FORMS   33

The 82 Forms of New-Style Tai Chi Ch'uan   34

First Sequence (Forms 1–20)   35

Second Sequence (Forms 21–40)   55

Third Sequence (Forms 41–60)   75

Fourth Sequence (Forms 61–82)   95

A Quick Review of New-Style Tai Chi Ch'uan Forms   117

INDEX   126

We would like to thank the many people who helped us with this book.
Our special thanks goes to Sung Kwan Ma, photography program,
the City College of the City University of New York,
for his painstaking work on the photographs.
His important contribution made this book possible.

UNDERSTANDING TAI CHI CH'UAN

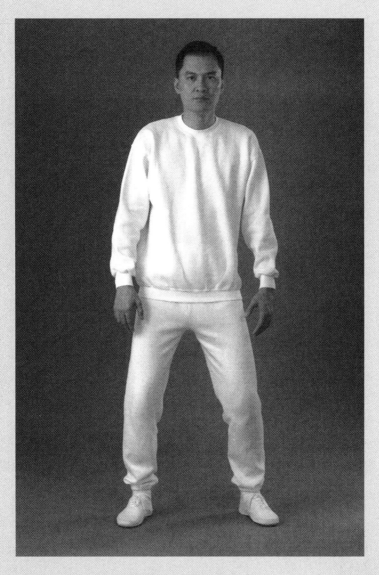

(1) Preparation, *Yu Pei Shih*. This is the beginning position for the first of 82 forms of New-Style Tai Chi Ch'uan.

For easy learning, we present four sequences, made up of about 20 forms each, with one or more movements per form. You'll find a complete list of the 82 forms on p. 34 and detailed instructions and photos for each form on pp. 35–116. To help you review the forms and sequences, you'll find a photo synopsis, "A Quick Review of New-Style Tai Chi Ch'uan Forms," on pp. 117–125.

The History of Tai Chi Ch'uan

Since the 1980s and 1990s in the United States and the Western world, newspaper and magazine articles, books, and movies have extolled the value of a centuries-old Chinese form of exercise, meditation, and self-defense known as tai chi ch'uan. Tai chi ch'uan is a moving form of meditation, and tai chi ch'uan's origins are closely related to those of meditation. In China, the practice of meditation began in prehistoric times. Its underlying principles can be found in the *I Ching,* or *Book of Changes,* written over 3,000 years ago.

Lao Tzu, the 6th century B.C. philosopher and one of the fathers of Taoism, developed theories basic to the traditional Chinese understanding of meditation, which in turn led to the development of tai chi ch'uan. The principles in his book, *Tao Te Ching,* deeply influenced later Taoist thought. Lao Tzu emphasized that "the soft overcomes the hard." In the centuries that followed, many Taoists developed these ideas into tai chi ch'uan and meditation.

In *Tao Te Ching,* Lao Tzu spoke in metaphors: "Can you keep the spirit and body without scattering?" This unity of spirit and body (or mind and body) is the fundamental idea of Taoist meditation. Taoists believe the body and mind must be united to achieve not simply longevity, but immortality.

"Can you concentrate your mind to use breath, making it as soft and quiet as an infant's?" The *breath* here is not just ordinary breath. First, it must become inner energy. Lao Tzu said that the respiration of ordinary people is from the throat and that true men of old breathed from the dantian and fully from their heels on up, not just from the abdomen. The dantian, commonly referred to by martial arts masters, is a point at the center of the body just 2 inches (5 cm) below the navel.

Infancy is the state in which the body is soft and pliant, and the mind quiet and innocent. The image of the infant also refers to the "holy fetus," which matures in meditation to emerge as the spirit infant. This recognition of the spirit infant within us is fundamental to tai chi ch'uan.

"Can you purify your contemplation and keep it from turbulence?" When one meditates, hundreds of thoughts sprout. We must clean away this turbulence, just as a mirror must be completely wiped free from dust in order to reflect purely.

After Lao Tzu, the second great master of Taoism was Chuang Tzu. His writings were entirely consistent with Lao Tzu's ideas, and he expressed them with clarity and expanded on them. Chuang Tzu also said that the breathing of the true man came deeply and silently, also explaining that the true man's breathing comes from his dantian and heels, while ordinary men usually breathe only from their throats. Many people, refusing to believe that the body can actually breathe through the dantian and heels, read this as a metaphor for some metaphysical idea. When considered in relation to the beginning of the first tai chi ch'uan form, *Yu Pei Shih,* or Preparation, however, the comment becomes clear.

At the beginning of form (1) *Yu Pei Shih,* or Preparation, the person practicing tai chi ch'uan stands with his feet firmly on the ground, directly below his shoulders. As he begins to inhale, his arms rise and his knees straighten. This lifts the vital energy from the ground upward through the heels, legs, and dantian. During the subsequent exhalation, his arms press downward and his knees bend, resulting in a lowering of the vital energy through the dantian, the legs, down to the heels, and back to the ground. The point is that in the practice of exercise and meditation, *breathing* refers not only to the movement of air in and out of the lungs, but to a process involving the whole body, including the circulation of oxygen to the extremities through the blood.

Chuang Tzu also wrote about this flow of vital energy through the body's channels. In his book, *Yang Sheng Chu,* he advised: "Use your mind to carry the vital energy along your channels upward constantly. This can keep your body healthy and your life long."

Tai chi ch'uan was not developed until centuries after Chuang Tzu lived. However, Chuang Tzu was aware of methods of exercise coordinated with breathing and meditation commonly practiced in his day, many of which may be considered ancestors of tai chi ch'uan. People in Chuang Tzu's time exercised "inhaling and exhaling the breath, expelling the old breath and taking in new," and they moved "like the sleeping bear," and "stretch[ed] and twist[ed] the neck like a bird." The attainment of longevity and health, Chuang Tzu explained, requires breathing, meditation, and movement. The bear and the bird evidently refer to movements from exercises well known to Chuang Tzu.

It was common for Chinese exercises to include movements adapted from those of animals and birds. There are several examples of this in tai chi ch'uan forms, which include movements such as Step Back and Drive the Monkey Away (*Tao Nien Hou*) and The White Crane Spreads Its Wings *(Bai He Liang Chi)*. The function of these movements is to guide breathing and circulation to help the vital energy flow through the body and have beneficial effects.

If movement represents tai chi ch'uan and stillness represents meditation, practicing them together is more efficient for the achievement of longevity. In another passage, "sitting and forgetting" is a way of freeing oneself from the body and the mind and becoming one with the infinite.

This passage makes clear that Chuang Tzu considered meditation to be a way of attaining a state of quietude and emptiness by following the Taoist idea of nonaction and nonbeing. Chuang Tzu lived during the Chin dynasty, which was later overthrown during the Warring States period, around 221 B.C.

For the next four centuries, China was ruled by the Han dynasty (202 B.C.–220 A.D.). This was a time of peace as well as creativity in science and the arts. In this era, the great philosopher Wei Po-Yang wrote his important book *Tsan Tung Chi,* which has been translated as *The Kinship of the Three, or the Accordance of the Book of Changes with the Phenomena of Composite Things.* In this book, Wei Po-Yang develops a method of meditation that's based on the *I Ching.* The book also considers alchemy and its uses.

He also compared the vital energy (chi) circulating through the body's channels, guided by the force of the mind or meditation, to the fundamental forces governing the universe on the largest scale. Thus, he described the processes of meditation in terms of the Taoist philosophy of yin and yang, and the body's channels. His idea that body processes reflect the same principles at work in the cosmos greatly influenced all later thinking about meditation.

Wei considered exercise with meditation important. He wrote: "You build a wall around the city so that the people will be safe." The idea of building a wall around a city (a practice common in ancient China as well as in Europe) represents the use of exercise to make the body strong and healthy (outside) and to prevent sickness (inside). The idea that "the people will be safe" suggests the peaceful mind inside a healthy body that allows the spirit to be active and able to achieve the concentration necessary for the successful practice of meditation.

In the 3rd century A.D., a surgeon, Hua To, invented an exercise called the Movement of the Five Animals. Hua To contributed additional movements of animals—the bear, tiger, monkey, deer, bird, and others—to the development of tai chi ch'uan. A series of eighteen forms of health exercises created by the alchemist Ko Hung (about 325 A.D.) completed the evolution of the Tao Yin. His work was discovered on a silk painting in an ancient tomb in Hunan province in 1974.

During the Han dynasty, Buddhism was introduced into China. By the 6th century A.D., Buddhism became as important as Taoism in Chinese religious and philosophical tradition. Buddhism had a direct influence on the development of meditation in China, since it brought its own traditional methods of meditation from India. Buddhists advocated the attainment of peace and tranquility by giving up desire and ridding oneself of the limited personal ego. As a means toward these ends, Buddhists used meditation.

The Shao Lin Method of Exercise

The invention of the Shao Lin Method of Exercise was an important development in the Buddhist meditation tradition. Master Ta Mo, who came to China from India around 530 A.D., established a school of Zen Buddhism in the Shao Lin monastery. While teaching meditation and Zen concepts to the monks, he became aware that his students were growing physically weaker. Their bodies were becoming as thin as dry wood, their faces turned pale, and many were sick.

Ta Mo thought a great deal about how to restore their health. According to legend, he sat in meditation facing a wall for nine years. The solution he finally discovered illustrates the fundamental philosophical principle that out of quietude grows movement. He developed a simple form of exercise to stimulate circulation, loosen the joints, and restore vitality. The monks soon found that regular practice of this exercise enabled them to meditate for long periods without undesirable physical effects.

Ta Mo and his followers later made the exercises more strenuous and systematic, and they also developed methods of boxing and using weapons such as knives and sticks. Thus the Shao Lin exercise became a system of martial arts. Shao Lin exercise also has many components similar to those found in tai chi ch'uan, such as meditation and breathing.

A similar development in the Taoist meditation tradition occurred several hundred years later. The great Taoist master Chang San-Feng, who was knowledgeable about the ancient wisdom of the *I Ching,* Confucianism, Buddhism, and Taoism, created, after a long period of meditation, the system of exercise known as tai chi ch'uan. His aim was similar to that of Ta Mo: to develop a form of discipline complementary to the practice of meditation that would also promote health. The resulting exercise method is different from that of Shao Lin, and it has quite distinct results.

Shao Lin's movements are generally strenuous and sometimes very quick. Regular practice of these forms strengthens the limbs and increases the size of the muscles. On the other hand, tai chi ch'uan movements are done slowly, gently, and evenly from beginning to end, each posture unfolding with the same continuous rhythm. This improves circulation and respiration and strengthens internal organs, but it does not increase muscle size. Because of this contrast, tai chi ch'uan is sometimes called the Inner School and Shao Lin the Outer School. In spite of these differences, both schools are, at their highest levels, forms of spiritual discipline, and both were originally developed to aid in the practice of meditation.

Shao Lin and tai chi ch'uan exercises eventually became known throughout China because of the many displays of self-defense skills by those who had become expert in their practice. Unfortunately, people often forget that these exercises were meant to aid meditation. People who were interested in self-defense came from far and wide to learn the exercises. Some wanted to use them for revenge. Others wanted to use them for military purposes. Still others wanted to create their own schools of martial arts or to teach the exercises in order to make a living.

Very few people had the patience or the single-mindedness necessary to learn meditation. In spite of this, the Buddhist and Taoist masters taught the exercises to many laymen, who in turn taught others for generation after generation.

Before long, many different schools and styles of self-defense exercises developed. However, most of the people who practiced them were unaware, and many remain unaware today, of the relationship between exercise and meditation.

Nevertheless, there is continuing evidence that meditation and exercise are each indispensable to the successful practice of the other. This is shown in the benefits of health, vigor, and longevity enjoyed by those who consciously practice both disciplines. It has also been found that in the experiences of masters, at the highest level, the two blend together automatically and unconsciously.

The famous master Yin Shih Tzu, who died in the mid-1980s in China, was enlightened in both Buddhist and Taoist meditation, which he had practiced for many years. He wrote a book about his experiences, *Yin Shih Tzu's Experimental Meditation for the Promotion of Health,* part of which has been translated into English by Lu Kuan Yu in his book *Secrets of Chinese Meditation.* In this book the master reported that he spent many years meditating and concentrating on opening the eight channels and twelve meridians to allow chi energy to flow through them. He finally achieved a state in which, feeling weightless and very warm, he suddenly noticed that his body was performing the tai chi ch'uan movements quite unconsciously and involuntarily. Dancers call this natural and effortless performance "muscle memory."

A contemporary Zen master, Huai Chin Nan, also studied Taoism in depth. He suggests using meditation and tai chi ch'uan together. In his book, Huai Chin Nan advocates that it is helpful for meditation to perform both tai chi ch'uan and chi kung.

Beijing Short-Form Tai Chi Ch'uan

The People's Republic of China was established in 1949, and later the Chinese National Physical Education Administration (CNPEA). When the CNPEA realized the need of a growing number of people wanting to learn tai chi ch'uan, they convened the first national workshop in 1970 in Beijing. Masters of different styles of tai chi ch'uan were invited from all over China to work together. With the aid of these experts, the CNPEA developed the first form of tai chi ch'uan to combine the different regional styles. They also made tai chi ch'uan easy to learn. This simplified tai chi ch'uan has 24 forms and is sometimes referred to as Beijing Short-Form Tai Chi Ch'uan.

The simplified or Beijing Short Form, accredited by the CNPEA, was taught across China in the 1970s and 1980s. It was thought to be a practical and simple way to learn the physical art. But many experts found drawbacks to the method. They thought it was not comprehensive enough to represent the different styles of tai chi ch'uan. This simplified method also focused more on physical movement while ignoring the elements of breathing, eye movement, and mental concentration integral to most martial arts. And this simplified method was also less useful for self-defense.

New-Style Tai Chi Ch'uan

So, the CNPEA convened another national workshop in 1988, inviting experts of the different styles in Anhui province to create a more comprehensive and beneficial tai chi ch'uan. From this workshop a new form of tai chi ch'uan called New-Style Tai Chi Ch'uan was developed that expanded the Beijing Short Form and incorporated additional movements from different regional styles of tai chi ch'uan.

People who had practiced the Beijing Short-Form Tai Chi Ch'uan and New-Style Tai Chi Ch'uan for years began to demand more comprehensive tai chi ch'uan movements that combined physical movements, meditation, breathing, eye movements, and self-defense. Based on this demand, the CNPEA convened the third national workshop in 1993 in Beijing, again inviting experts of different styles from all over China and from other countries. The CNPEA created a more comprehensive New-Style Tai Chi Ch'uan, which will be presented in this book. It is intended to satisfy masters, students, and novices alike.

Of course, each tai chi ch'uan master has his or her own expression of the art. This 1993 official Chinese system, used in physical education classes across China, necessarily bears our imprint, as it will yours when you make it your own.

The Philosophy of Tai Chi Ch'uan
Yin & Yang

The philosophical theory behind the practice of tai chi ch'uan is based on the Tao as a coming together of opposites. The two opposing manifestations of the Tao, called yin and yang, have universal significance and apply to the phenomena of the cosmos as well as to the operations of the human body. On the largest scale, heaven is yang, while earth is yin. Day is yang, while night is yin. Bright and clear weather is yang; dark and stormy weather is yin. On the scale of living things, the male is yang and the female is yin. Spirit is yang and body is yin.

This opposition also applies to the parts of the body and their functions. In the circulatory system, the arteries are yang and the veins are yin. In breathing, exhalation is yang and inhalation is yin. In human activities, movement is yang and rest is yin.

A systematic description of the relationships of yin and yang is found in the hexagrams of the *I Ching,* the oldest and most important book of Chinese philosophy. The hexagrams themselves were developed in ancient China and date to more than two centuries before the philosopher and physician Huang Ti. His health practices, consisting of an alternation of movement and rest, and his form of exercise involving breathing in and out were direct applications of the yin and yang principle.

This principle of opposites, or dualism, has been the basis of the Chinese understanding of health and sickness since ancient times. Good health requires a balance between yin and yang forces within the body. If either one or the other is too predominant, sickness results, and it is the aim of the medical sciences, including acupuncture and herbal medicine, to discover the source of the imbalance and restore the forces to their proper proportion, or harmony.

However, the Taoist philosophy that underlies the practice of tai chi ch'uan and meditation involves a somewhat more complex theory of the relationship between yin and yang within the body. Taoism does not deny that a general balance between these forces is necessary to avoid sickness. Nevertheless, in certain respects, it is the aim of tai chi ch'uan to greatly increase the yang and to reduce and diminish the yin.

One of the fundamental beliefs of Taoist philosophy is that the reason people become old and weak and eventually die is that they lack sexual energy. This explanation is based on the insight that physical reproduction is but one aspect of the process of maintaining the life and creativity of the individual person. When we are young, our sexual activities naturally generate a powerful energy that pervades all aspects of life, both physical and mental. The generation of this energy occurs in the production of sexual essences: the sperm in the male and the menstrual fluid in the female. These substances are both yang. As we grow old and these essences are no longer produced so easily, this natural source of energy tends to dwindle and become less powerful. Thus the sexual essence can be thought of as somewhat like the fuel in a machine. When the machine runs out of fuel, it can no longer move.

However, such a loss of energy is not an inevitable result of growing old. Since ancient times, Taoist philosophy has been concerned with the question of how to reproduce and maintain this kind of energy so as to prolong the life and creativity of the individual. The answer to the question is to be found in the methods of tai chi ch'uan. In tai chi ch'uan, a combination of movements, breathing, and mental concentration (meditation) is used to purify the sexual essence, distilling its pure yang aspect (vital energy, or chi) and transmitting chi through the eight channels and twelve meridians to every cell in the body.

The ultimate aim of such methods, according to classic Taoist treatises, is nothing short of the attainment of physical immortality. Taoism has long carried the conviction that this is actually possible. The regular practice of tai chi ch'uan has definitely been shown to result in longevity, good health, vigor, mental alertness, and creativity far beyond what is experienced by most people. In fact, it can also greatly prolong sexual potency and activity.

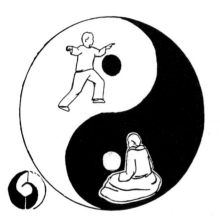

Yin and Yang
Tai Chi Tu, the Supreme Ultimate

Traditional *Tai Chi Tu* Diagram

To obtain full benefit from practicing tai chi ch'uan, it is essential to understand Taoist philosophy and the principles of yin and yang. The practices of tai chi ch'uan, meditation, and breathing should complement one another. The relationship between them manifests itself as a subtle interweaving of opposite (yin and yang) tendencies.

Observe the *Tai Chi Tu* diagram of the "supreme ultimate" with two fishlike figures within a circle: one black, one white (see above). The white "fish," representing movement, is called the "greater yang." Within each figure is a smaller circle of the opposite color, which may be seen as the "eye" of the fish. The black circle within the white figure is called the "lesser yin," and the white circle within the black "fish" is called the "lesser yang." These inner circles represent the way each of the opposing forces, yin and yang, contains within itself its opposite and continuously originates from its opposite in a smooth, never-ending cycle.

The Yin & Yang of Tai Chi Ch'uan

In the practice of tai chi ch'uan, the relationship between movement and rest should reflect the interweaving of yang and yin represented in the diagram. Tai chi ch'uan, essentially a form of movement, is yang, the white fish. Meditation, which involves the mind or imagination quietly, is yin, the black fish. Breathing combines both yin and yang with exhalation (yang) and inhalation (yin). But this distinction takes into account only the external aspects of these activities.

To perform tai chi ch'uan correctly, one must be very peaceful and quiet inside (yin) while executing the externally visible movements (yang). The practitioner must use mental concentration and breath to move chi, his vital energy, through the body's channels and meridians while remaining still. Thus the inner aspect of the practice is opposite to its outer aspect, just as the greater yang contains the lesser yin within it and vice versa.

Seen in yet another way, the diagram represents the way in which movement and meditation grow out of each other as alternating practices. The movements of tai chi ch'uan, while producing more and more energy and vitality, tend to increase the yang side of the yin-yang balance in the body. Eventually, when the yang reaches a high point, it generates a need to be quiet and to purify energy. This is done through meditation, which produces a more peaceful condition, increasing the yin side of the balance. When the yin reaches a high point, it generates a need to increase the yang once again.

Through this alternating practice of two opposite methods, combined with breathing, one can obtain beneficial effects, including longevity. Yin alternates with yang just as inhaling (passive yin) must be followed by exhaling (active yang) to promote the health and the life of both body and mind. So, too, in life one must alternate yin and yang activities to live long and to prosper.

The Physiology of Tai Chi Ch'uan
The Channels & Meridians

To learn the disciplines of meditation and tai chi ch'uan successfully, it helps to know the basic physiological foundation of tai chi ch'uan: channels and meridians.

This requirement is analogous to the idea that one cannot easily develop athletic skills without being aware of the body processes through the study of anatomy and physiology. Tai chi ch'uan meditation involves the circulation of chi, or energy, throughout the body. To experience this circulation, it is helpful to have a notion of the location of specific points and the pathways or channels between these points along which the energy flows.

The traditional Chinese concept of the human body differs somewhat from the Western one. The most notable difference is that Chinese physiological descriptions make use of terms and ideas that Westerners regard as spiritual or psychological. For example, *chi,* or vital energy, does not refer to any physical entity that can be readily detected or measured with scientific instruments. It is an invisible substance that can only be felt *inside* the body as it flows through the channels and meridians. The eight channels inside the body and the twelve meridians that run along the surface of the body are likewise invisible and cannot be detected by usual physical methods. The Western scientific mind, which tends to view the body as a biochemical machine, is likely to regard such concepts with considerable skepticism.

However, these concepts are important to Chinese thought since they are essential to the theory of meditation and to the theory of the highly sophisticated Chinese medical practices of acupuncture and acupressure, as well as tai chi ch'uan and chi kung.

The Eight Channels

Eight connective pathways that both transmit and store energy are located in the trunk of the body and in the head, arms, and legs. Through them, energy can reach every cell in the body. The method of systematically circulating chi through these channels involves practicing meditation while practicing tai chi ch'uan. The eight channels are (1) *Tu Mo* (control), (2) *Jen Mo* (function), (3) *Tai Mo* (belt), (4) *Cheung Mo* (thrusting), (5) *Yang Yu Wei Mo* (positive arm), (6) *Yin Yu Wei Mo* (negative arm), (7) *Yang Chiao Mo* (positive leg), and (8) *Yin Chiao Mo* (negative leg). See descriptions below and diagrams on p. 16.

Tu Mo (**Control Channel**) runs along the spinal column, beginning at the coccyx, continuing up through the neck to the skull, and over the crown of the head to the roof of the mouth.

Jen Mo (**Function Channel**) goes through the center and front of the body. It begins at the genitals and extends up to the base of the mouth. When the tongue rests against the palate, it forms a bridge between the *tu mo* and the *jen mo* channels.

Tai Mo (**Belt Channel**) circles the waist like a belt. It begins under the navel and divides into two branches, which extend around the waist to the small of the back.

Cheung Mo (**Thrusting Channel**) passes through the center of the body in front of the *tu mo* and behind the *jen mo* channels. Its begins at the genitals and extends upward, ending just below the heart.

The Eight Channels

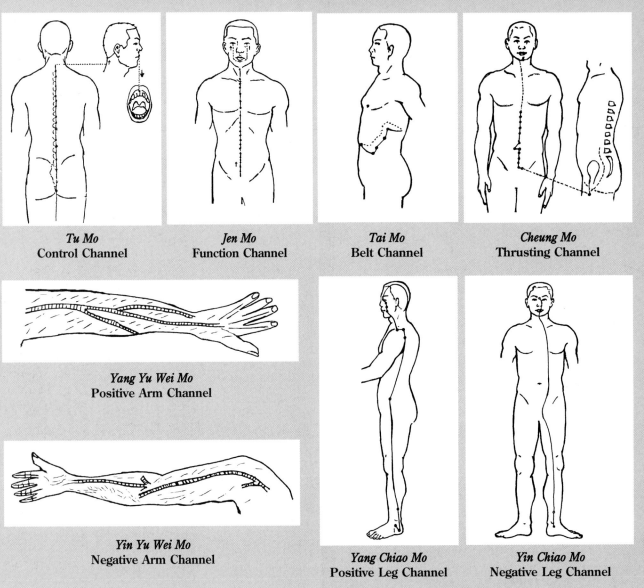

Tu Mo
Control Channel

Jen Mo
Function Channel

Tai Mo
Belt Channel

Cheung Mo
Thrusting Channel

Yang Yu Wei Mo
Positive Arm Channel

Yin Yu Wei Mo
Negative Arm Channel

Yang Chiao Mo
Positive Leg Channel

Yin Chiao Mo
Negative Leg Channel

Yang Yu Wei Mo (**Positive Arm Channel**) begins below the navel, passes through the chest to the shoulders, down the outside of the arms to the middle fingertips, then around to the center of the palms.

Yin Yu Wei Mo (**Negative Arm Channel**) extends inside the arms from the palms to the shoulders, ending in the chest.

Yang Chiao Mo (**Positive Leg Channel**) extends along both sides of the body, from the center of the soles of the feet, outside the ankles and legs, up to the head, finally ending below the ears. The bilateral beginnings of this channel, located in the soles, are called *yung ch'uan* cavities.

The Chinese term *yung ch'uan* means "bubbling spring."

Yin Chiao Mo **(Negative Leg Channel)** also begins in the *yung ch'uan* cavities. It then extends up through the inside of the legs, to the genitals, up the center of the body, and ends at a point between the eyebrows.

Together the eight channels form an interconnected network through which chi can flow freely inside the body during meditation.

The Twelve Meridians

In addition to the channels within the body, there are twelve energy pathways at the surface of the body, called *meridians.* These are connected to the internal organs by intermediate circulatory paths. The twelve meridians take their names from the specific internal organs to which they correspond.

Acupuncture and acupressure can help regulate and balance the distribution of energy within the internal organs by manipulating key points that lie along these twelve meridians. There are about 700 acupuncture or acupressure points. Of these, there are three main types: (1) *tonification points,* through which energy can be increased when there is a deficiency; (2) *sedation points,* through which energy can be decreased when there is an excess; and (3) *source points.*

Each meridian has a fixed direction, called either *centrifugal* (away from the center of the body or the dantian) or *centripetal* (toward the center of the body or the dantian). In addition, each is designated as either yin or yang, depending on the character of the energy that flows along it. (See pp. 12–14 for understanding yin and yang energy.) They are bilateral. See p. 18 for diagrams for each of these twelve meridians: (1) lung, (2) kidney, (3) large intestine, (4) spleen, (5) gallbladder, (6) triple warmer, (7) heart, (8) bladder, (9) stomach, (10) small intestine, (11) heart governor, and (12) liver.

Lung Meridian *(yin; centrifugal)* runs along the sides of the body. It begins between the second and third ribs near the armpits, goes up to the shoulders, runs down the arms, and ends at the base of the thumbnails.

Kidney Meridian *(yin; centripetal)* begins on the soles of the feet, goes up the inside of the legs to the center of the body, just above the genitals, and runs along the chest, ending between the collarbone and first ribs.

Large Intestine Meridian *(yang; centripetal)* begins at the base of the nail of the index fingers, travels along the arms up to the shoulders and neck, and ends just beside the nostrils.

Spleen Meridian *(yin; centripetal)* begins at the root of the nail of the big toes, goes up along the inside of the legs and the sides of the torso, and ends below the armpits.

Gallbladder Meridian *(yang; centrifugal)* begins at the outside corner of the eyes, passes through several points on the head, goes down the sides of the body and legs, and ends at the second joint of the fourth toes.

Triple Warmer Meridian *(yang; centrifugal)* begins on the outer side of the ring fingers (toward the little fingers) and travels up the hands and arms to the head, ending just below the eyebrows.

Heart Meridian *(yin; centrifugal)* begins inside the armpits and runs down the inner side of the arms to the base of the little fingers.

Bladder Meridian *(yang; centrifugal)* begins on the inside corner of the eyes, goes up over the top of the skull, down the back near the spine, down the back of the legs, and ends at the base of the nail on the little toes.

Stomach Meridian *(yin; centrifugal)* begins under the eyes and moves down the chest and abdomen, along the front of the legs to the base of the second toenails.

The Twelve Meridians

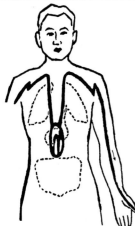

Lung Meridian

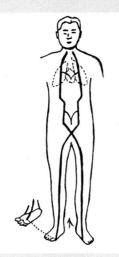

Kidney Meridian

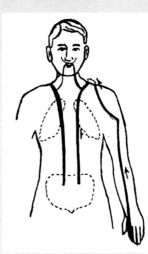

Large Intestine Meridian

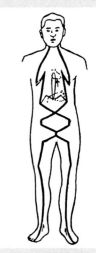

Spleen Meridian

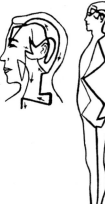

Gallbladder Meridian

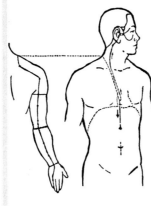

Triple Warmer Meridian

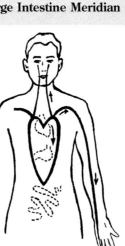

Heart Meridian

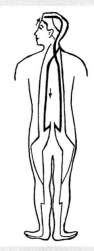

Bladder Meridian

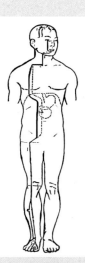

Stomach Meridian

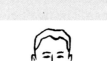

Small Intestine Meridian

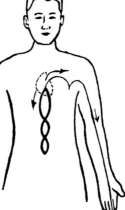

Heart Governor Meridian

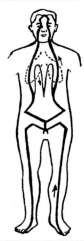

Liver Meridian

Small Intestine Meridian *(yang; centripetal)* begins at the base of the little fingernails, runs up the arms to the sides of the neck, then around to the front of the face, and finally back over to the front of the ears.

Heart Governor Meridian *(yin; centrifugal)* begins on the chest and travels down the arms and hands to the base of the middle fingernails.

Liver Meridian *(yin; centripetal)* begins at the base of the large toenails and extends up the legs and abdomen to the chest near the nipples.

Detecting Channels & Meridians

Channels and meridians are the physiological foundation of tai chi ch'uan. When we practice tai chi ch'uan, meditation directs the chi, or vital energy, to circulate within the body's channels and meridians in coordination with breathing and physical movements.

Western scientists have dissected the body in an attempt to find the channels and meridians—the pathways along which chi flows—but they have had no real success. Yet Western doctors have seen acupuncturists "cure" apparently incurable diseases. About 700 points on the surface of these pathways seem to mark key points in the body's physiology and pathology used in traditional Chinese medicine. Acupuncture, which uses these points, channels, and meridians, seems to work, even though it is not yet clear how.

Since the 1970s, many European physicians and physical therapists have begun using acupuncture in their treatments. After Nixon's visit to China in 1972, many Americans, Canadians, and other Westerners have visited or studied in China and accepted the concept of Chinese traditional medicine. With the growing news coverage, the Western world has renewed interest in the medical possibilities of acupuncture. Most Western physicians have tended to focus on the use of acupuncture as an "anesthetic" in both major and minor surgery.

Dissection of cadavers, however, may not be the best way to determine whether chi and its pathways (channels and meridians) actually exist. This vital energy apparently ceases to flow after death.

In 1939 in the north Caucasian town of Krasnodar, an Armenian electrician named Semyon Davidovich Kirlian discovered a photographic method that uses high-frequency electrical fields to record on film the energy coming from the human body and from plants. Some years later, Dr. Mikhail Kuzmich Gaikin, a Leningrad surgeon, read about Kirlian's work. He was reminded of the explanation for acupuncture learned from Chinese doctors during his army service in China. He went to see Kirlian.

As Gaikin and Kirlian looked at photographs of a human body under high-frequency electrical fields, they found that the spots where lights flared most brilliantly appeared to match the acupuncture points the Chinese had mapped thousands of years ago! Gaikin was excited. They supposed this discovery might provide the first scientific confirmation of the 5,000-year-old practice of Chinese medicine, acupuncture. They speculated that there could also be a relationship between the pathways of swimming light revealed in these photographs of a human body and the channels and meridians of vital energy, or chi, described by the ancient Chinese.

After studying the Kirlian process, Dr. Gaikin, in collaboration with an engineer, Vladislov Mikalevsky, developed the *tobiscope,* an electronic device that locates the points on the body into which acupuncture needles are inserted. These points are less than 1 millimeter wide and traditionally have been difficult to pinpoint accurately. The tobiscope could locate the position of the acupuncture points within 0.1 millimeter.

Research by Kirlian, Gaikin, Mikalevsky, and others suggests that the chi described by many ancient tai chi ch'uan masters may be more than a poetic indulgence or an effort to imbue their art with magic.

Kirlian photography, also known as bioelectrography, could do what other advanced medical tools and devices could not. Even modern diagnostic tools, like the CAT scan, MRI, and PET scan, used to image the body's activities and structure, fail to reveal the body's channels and meridians as well as the 700 points important in acupuncture.

The CAT (computed axial tomography), or simply CT, scan uses X rays to record a series of cross-sectional images of the body. The MRI (magnetic resonance imaging), based on nuclear magnetic resonance of atoms within the body induced by radio waves, reveals computerized images of internal body structures. The PET (positron emission tomography) scan uses radioactive particles and the metabolic rate to evaluate activity of specific brain tissue.

Today many Western naturopathic physicians use Kirlian photography, or bioelectrography, as a method of interpretation for medical diagnosis. They usually analyze the corona of the fingertips in relation to their function as endpoints of the meridians of traditional Chinese medicine, acupressure and acupuncture, and Japanese shiatsu or acupressure (finger massage of acupuncture points). Naturopathic physicians may also apply German neo-acupuncture to their analysis.

This research helps validate the theory that when we practice tai chi ch'uan correctly, in a relaxed way with meditation and directed breathing, we open the pathways along which this vital chi energy flows. Opening these pathways may help *correct imbalances in this energy flow*—with consequent benefits to our health.

Meditation

The Flow of Chi through Channels & Meridians

Learning to relax physically is one way tension-ridden people attempt to find peace and tranquility. Some have turned to alcohol, nicotine, or other drugs to slow racing mental and emotional engines, and they have found that these drugs have harmful side effects. Others have chosen various kinds of meditation to relieve stress.

Sitting Meditation & Moving Meditation

Tai chi ch'uan, in addition to conferring health benefits related to exercise, can be thought of as "moving meditation." Many people who have done "sitting meditation" alone, in an effort to achieve tranquility, have been strongly impressed by how helpful tai chi ch'uan can be in achieving this goal.

Practitioners consider moving meditation philosophically satisfying because everything in the universe is in constant motion, and they believe they can best harmonize with the universe through a meditation that also moves. People who are attracted by Taoism, Buddhism, and Confucianism find in tai chi ch'uan a physical expression of the principles expounded in these Chinese philosophies. Whatever a practitioner's reason for meditating—whether to relieve mental tension or to achieve spiritual enlightenment—meditation can have mind-quieting and mind-expanding results.

Tai chi ch'uan is ideally suited for meditation because, when correctly performed, we must give it our full attention. We should not entertain extraneous thoughts and ideas that may intrude as we are practicing a particular tai chi ch'uan form. The mind must immediately return to focus completely on the correct performance of the movement, the way we meditate, and the breathing. We gradually become able to concentrate fully on meditation, breathing, and movement for longer periods without becoming distracted by problems or irrelevant thoughts.

Practicing tai chi ch'uan as meditation can provide a period of quiet calm that's necessary for all of us. It is especially helpful for maintaining mental equilibrium in the stressful conditions of modern life. If we spend a part of each day in an activity that relaxes us mentally and physically, this allows us to pull scattered thoughts together. It also removes us from interaction with others. This practice renews us and enables us to face responsibilities with additional strength. Through the weeks, months, and years we can develop a direct and relaxed approach to difficult tasks that allows us to complete them relatively quickly.

Unlike other kinds of meditation (sitting or standing), tai chi ch'uan, as a moving meditation, uses arm and leg movements to coordinate the meditation, inner concentration, and breathing that guide the chi through the body's channels and meridians. Although tai chi ch'uan forms and movements are not very complicated, when combined with meditation they very effectively direct the circulation of chi's refining energy through these pathways. Common tai chi ch'uan movements—like shifting your weight from one leg to another, rotating the body to the right or left, taking a step, moving forward or backward, and various hand and foot movements—when coordinated with meditation help both body and mind.

The roles of the mind and the chi are even more important than the movements themselves. In tai chi ch'uan it is usually said: "The mind directs the chi and the chi mobilizes the body." The mind indeed guides the chi to every part of the body, including the smallest cells, cavities, joints, and bones. During certain movements the chi may have several destinations. For example, in the forms (52–55) Fair Lady Weaving at the Shuttle I–IV *(Yu Nu Ch'uan Sho)*, the chi may circulate through and around the torso, or the mind may direct the chi all the way to the fingers and toes.

While the outer movements (like crossing the arms) remain the same, the inner movements (circulation) of chi may be directed farther and deeper. The mind also directs the breathing, important to both tai chi ch'uan and meditation, since the outside breath helps form the vital chi energy directed by meditation. All "outside" tai chi ch'uan movements described in this book should be coordinated with meditation and chi movement "inside." When practicing tai chi ch'uan, we should imagine and guide the chi movement within the channels and meridians with meditation.

Breathing
The Exercise of Yin & Yang

In China, breathing has been an important subject of study for over 5,000 years. Taoists have used breathing techniques to prevent sickness, prolong youth, achieve longevity, and ultimately to reach their highest goal, immortality. Many schools of tai chi ch'uan use breathing to exercise yin and yang and to coordinate meditation and chi (vital energy) circulation within the body's channels and meridians.

In recent years, Western interest in these breathing techniques has grown. Many physicians are aware that deep breathing can preserve health and cure diseases, but they do not understand the secret of combining breathing, yin and yang, meditation, chi, and physical movements. Although many Western books and periodicals have dealt with this, scientific analysis of breathing techniques, including that essential to tai chi ch'uan, has lagged behind.

However, many ideas have been proposed through the years. Besides oxygen, the air that we breathe contains many elements, including iron, copper, zinc, fluorite, quartz, zincite, and magnesium. These elements supply important bodily needs. By using a combination of tai chi ch'uan meditation, physical movement, and breathing, Taoist techniques provide an efficient method for taking in these precious elements and getting rid of wastes and toxins. These techniques, as tai chi ch'uan masters say, "expel the old; take in the new."

According to Buddhists and Taoists, the body is a "dirty leather bag" because it contains all kinds of things—toxins, wastes, impaired bone, and old tissue. The breath can clean this dirty bag when properly used and guided by meditation and chi movement within the channels and meridians.

Prenatal & Postnatal Breathing

Taoist and Buddhist breathing techniques include not only mouth and nose breathing, but also fetal, or internal, breathing. The concepts of prenatal breathing and postnatal breathing appear in Taoist writings and diagrams. Taoists explain that before birth the embryo does not need to inhale and exhale, since the breath is circulated through the body from the mother. Oxygen-rich blood comes into the body through the umbilical cord and enters the abdomen at the navel.

Thus, prenatal breathing is done through the abdomen. After birth, of course, this method of breathing is no longer available since the umbilical cord is severed. Thereafter, the baby, child, and adult must rely on breathing through the lungs: postnatal breathing. Most people only breathe with the throat and lungs, so that the prenatal breath "hides" in the abdomen, never again joining the postnatal breath.

However, this prenatal capability plays a role in the practice of tai chi ch'uan and meditation. So meditation and tai chi ch'uan may be said to unite prenatal and postnatal breathing. That is, during inhalation, as the meditator is drawing the postnatal breath into the lungs and down to the navel (dantian), the prenatal breath rises up from the lower abdomen to the navel, where it joins the postnatal breath to achieve the goal of exercising the yin. During exhalation, as the postnatal breath rises up out of the lungs or moves out from the upper or lower extremities, the prenatal breath sinks down again to the lower abdominal region to achieve the goal of exercising the yang.

In very advanced stages of meditation and tai chi ch'uan, there is a phenomenon called fetal breathing in which the person meditating, like the embryo, is able to breathe without inhaling and exhaling. In this stage, which is also characterized by an absence of pulse, the meditator completely transcends conscious thought and attains a state called Great Quiescence. This is the highest form of enlightenment and the ultimate goal of tai chi ch'uan meditation.

Tai chi ch'uan experts believe that everyone is in the air and the air is inside everyone. In heaven as well as on earth nearly all creatures depend on air. The true practitioner of tai chi ch'uan meditation and breathing fortifies his body inside and protects it from outside harm. The outside air is, of course, the atmosphere of the earth. The air inside the body is oxygen and prenatal or fetal breathing. Everyone recognizes the importance of oxygen, but very few people are aware of prenatal breathing. When a person dies a natural death, it is thought that prenatal breathing has become exhausted. Buddhists and Taoists say, "When the oil is finished, the lamp is black." Tai chi ch'uan's meditative breathing appears to increase the oil inside the lamp so that it will continue to burn for decades. In other words, it will help promote longevity.

Great tai chi ch'uan masters use the power of chi combined with breathing. They advise practitioners preparing to attack to inhale and store the chi in the abdomen (dantian) guided by meditation, like drawing a bow. When attacking, they exhale and release chi from the abdomen (dantian), like shooting the arrow.

When Master Yang Chien Hou (1842–1917) was in the courtyard, the story is told, he let his student punch him in the abdomen. As the student did so, the tai chi ch'uan master suddenly let out the laughing sound "Ha!" The student fell back twenty steps—so strong was the power of the chi released through this sound.

The chi must be accumulated gradually and slowly through meditation and breathing. Tai chi ch'uan masters compare it to the wind. "So it is with the accumulation of wind: if it be not great, it will not have the strength to support great wings." From a small breeze the wind gradually becomes a tornado. The small breeze cannot move the weak grass. But when the breeze increases to become a tornado, it can uproot trees, hurl houses into space, and knock down tall buildings.

To accumulate chi in the body through practicing meditation and breathing, constant, regular, and unhurried practice of tai chi ch'uan is required. Tai chi ch'uan masters say: "Let not the mind forget its work, but let there be no assisting the growth of that nature." Such practice should never try to force results.

Let us not be like the man from the village of Sung. A man from Sung was grieved that his growing corn was not longer, so he pulled it up. After doing this, he returned home, looking very stupid, and said to his family: "I am tired today. I have been helping the corn to grow long." His son ran to look at it and found the corn lying on the ground, all withered.

The Physical Movements of Tai Chi Ch'uan

Extravagant claims have been made for the health-promoting and health-restoring qualities of tai chi ch'uan. What legitimate claims can be made for tai chi ch'uan as physical exercise? In general, people who do exercise regularly have better circulation, better muscle tone, and fewer illnesses than people who do not exercise. In addition, those who exercise usually enjoy a feeling of physical and mental well-being.

Most writers on fitness concern themselves with the effect of regular exercise on the heart and circulatory system. They generally share the conclusion that if we are to remain in good health, the heart must be given work beyond the minimal demands made on it by sedentary living. Recommended exercises often include jogging, swimming, tennis, golf, skiing, and more. But these exercises are not suitable for people of all age groups and fitness levels. Walking and tai chi ch'uan, milder and less strenuous forms of exercise, are usually recommended for older people, people in poor health, or those recovering from an illness.

The Gentle Exercise

When considered strictly as a fitness-producing exercise, how does tai chi ch'uan compare with an activity like jogging or swimming? Tai chi ch'uan is an ideal way to exercise for people interested in attaining and maintaining physical fitness but for whom a high level of athletic fitness is unnecessary. Because tai chi ch'uan does not include extreme movements and emphasizes gradual learning, practitioners avoid the pulled muscles and other injuries that sometimes accompany more strenuous activities. Practitioners are not called upon to twist and turn in a way that might cause body parts to suffer strain. Instead, tai chi ch'uan encourages a feeling of restraint, with no forced movement.

Some sports and exercises combine maximum range of movement with maximum speed, a combination that can injure the body. A tennis or golf swing performed when we begin playing without a proper warm-up can cause pulled or torn muscles. The possibility of such injury increases when we only exercise on weekends rather than three or four times a week. Experts agree that weekend-only exercise is a dangerous practice because the body, unaccustomed to demands, will react adversely instead of being helped. Tai chi ch'uan requires no special equipment, can be practiced in the living room, and is well suited as daily exercise.

Leg Work

Those who begin to practice tai chi ch'uan soon realize that, though the exercise is gentle, it is *not* effortless. Tai chi ch'uan demands considerable work by the leg muscles because it is done with bent knees in a kind of quarter squat. Weight shifts from foot to foot as we do a particular form, but we do not stand fully erect until the last form is completed. As we improve, we find we are able to sink lower in individual forms. This process gradually strengthens the legs and increases their muscle tone.

It's best to wait until after a knee injury has healed before attempting tai chi ch'uan. Many people continue to feel pain or discomfort months or even years after recovery from the initial injury. Tai chi ch'uan can be helpful at this time, because it helps strengthen leg muscles and thereby support the knee(s). In any case, it is best to consult a physician before resuming normal physical activities and exercise.

Better leg development is beneficial to the body's health in a number of ways. Experts on cardiovascular fitness emphasize that firm, strong leg muscles are very important in aiding circulation. The heart benefits from the pumping action of the muscles of the extremities, particularly those of the legs. When leg muscles contract and squeeze veins in the legs, the valves in these veins prevent the blood from going away from the heart. Thus, the pull of gravity in the body's upright position is counteracted by good muscle tone and activity in the legs, and more blood is directed to the heart to be passed on, in turn, to the brain and other vital tissues.

Interest & Variety in Exercise

If people are to exercise regularly, month after month and year after year—a requirement that fitness experts consider important for continued good health—they must have an exercise they find interesting. For many people, calisthenics become boring. Running laps around a track or swimming from one end to another of a pool often becomes mentally tiresome. Some people enjoy jogging over changing terrain, but weather conditions sometimes prohibit this form of exercise.

Few activities can match the varied movements of tai chi ch'uan, which are based on self-defense techniques. Because practitioners must attend to meditation, breathing, balance, and coordination, they cannot do the forms automatically. It is important that the performance and movements absorb our attention. People usually derive less than optimum benefit from doing exercise they consider boring.

Relaxation & Stress Reduction

Learning to relax contributes to a more efficient use of the body, but it confers benefits beyond this. Tai chi ch'uan emphasizes relaxation. As we do individual forms, muscles not needed are kept loose and free of tension. Shoulders are not raised or tightened, and the chest is not thrown forward or out. Breathing becomes deeper, and the stomach can move in and out with each breath. Finally, the hands and wrists are never tensed in these exercises. The aim, however, is not slackness or collapse, but an alert relaxation, which can respond in an instant to some external threat.

Most people who are aware of their own physical tension also notice that they are mentally tense. Often mental and emotional tension manifest themselves physically. Many city dwellers search for a measure of tranquility in their lives. Researchers have found that lost tranquility and increasing tension are chief causes of heart disease and other major illnesses.

People who share certain personality traits— the hard-driving, highly competitive people (type A personality)—are more susceptible to stress than individuals who have an easygoing attitude toward life (type B personality). Anger or hostility, more common to type A personalities, can exacerbate stress and its effects on the body. If one is stress-prone or has type A behavior, what can be done to reduce stress or to counter its injurious effects? Many scientists seeking ways to reduce the harmful effects of stress have begun to recommend tai chi ch'uan.

Aid in Energy Flow

It may be profitable to examine tai chi ch'uan's contribution to health from still another standpoint. Doctors of Chinese medicine often refer to chi, a life force or vital energy that flows through the body on channels and meridians guided by meditation.

This vital energy can be tapped at over 700 points on the body where the channels and meridians come to the surface. Acupuncture uses these points to correct any imbalance in the energy flow that has adversely affected organ function. Tai chi ch'uan movements, coordinated with meditation and breathing, aid this vital energy flow through the body's channels and meridians.

The Health Benefits of Tai Chi Ch'uan

The purpose of practicing tai chi ch'uan is to improve health and prolong life. Elements or conditions inside the body threaten health, and therefore longevity, more seriously than do outside agents or injuries. These conditions can become dangerous, even life-threatening, because people often underestimate them.

Those who suffer from illnesses of the body's internal organs feel only minor discomfort at first. Many put off consulting a physician until the disease has reached a critical stage. By this time, it is often too late to correct the disease without costly medicines or invasive surgery. Severe illnesses of these organs may prove fatal. The expense—money, time, and suffering—that results from physical disorders can be minimized or avoided through the practice of tai chi ch'uan.

We need to identify the source of diseases. Not taking care of oneself means that the body's resistance to bacteria and viruses is diminished. Microbes can then attack the intestines, heart, pancreas, liver, and other organs more easily. Tuberculosis, stomach ulcers, and breast cancer are but a few of many diseases that infect the body's internal organs.

Tai chi ch'uan may help prevent such diseases. Our objectives are: (1) to keep the internal organs clean and free of acute or degenerative disorders, and (2) if these disorders are already present, to remove them.

For centuries Chinese medicine has recognized both the mental and physical aspects of disease. Traditionally, the mental state of the patient was considered to be even more important than his physical symptoms. Recently, a new field of Western medical research, *psychoneuro-immunology,* the study of the effect of emotions on disease, has emerged. Studies indicate that virtually every illness from the common cold to cancer and heart disease can be influenced, positively or negatively, by one's mental state. Today Western physicians and mental-health professionals are increasingly recognizing the role of the mind in the prevention and cure of disease.

Tai chi ch'uan includes specific techniques for attaining peaceful mental states that can help prevent and cure sickness. Tai chi ch'uan integrates the body and mind (meditation), breathing and movement, arms and legs, hands and feet. Integrated, the whole body can move as one. The mind is used to direct the vital energy or chi and to move the limbs of the body. The movement propels the blood throughout the system. This circulation helps the functioning of the internal organs.

Benefits for the Lungs

Meditation, as well as the open and closed movements of tai chi ch'uan, are coordinated with breathing. This action resembles that of bellows. The lungs are never at rest. Even in sleep, they continue to work. The deep breathing produced by tai chi ch'uan draws the breath down into the dantian, putting less pressure on the lungs, which get a chance to rest. When he was young, a famous tai chi ch'uan teacher, Zhang Ming, had coughed up blood and discovered he had tuberculosis. As he learned tai chi ch'uan, eventually becoming a master, his body was cured of the tuberculosis virus.

Benefits for the Heart

Heart disease is extremely prevalent in the United States. It is the most frequent cause of death. The deep breathing produced by tai chi ch'uan helps prevent and cure this illness. By using the mind to direct the movement of the limbs and to regulate breathing, chi is produced.

Chi helps the blood circulate, which reduces the workload on the heart. Improvement of the circulation that results from chi flowing within the body's channels and meridians, guided by meditation, will, for instance, help remove a clot, or thrombus, within the blood vessels. Tai chi ch'uan can *prevent* heart disease, and it can also *cure* and *rehabilitate* the heart patient.

Benefits for the Liver

The liver is as important to the body as the heart and the lungs. It secretes bile, changes sugar into glycogen, and affects the immune system. If the liver ceases to function properly, serious illness can result. Many liver diseases develop from viral infections and toxins deposited inside the body. Practicing tai chi ch'uan can, on the one hand, improve immune-system function, which in turn can prevent and cure viral infection. On the other hand, tai chi ch'uan—through meditation, breathing, and flowing chi—can clean and remove the deposited toxins.

Benefits for the Kidneys

The ancient Taoists spoke of the kidneys as the source of life. If the kidneys are weak, the body is weak. If the kidneys are not functioning properly, one will always feel tired and be sexually impotent.

In Taoist terminology, the kidneys are referred to as the moon and water, and the heart as the sun and fire. When water and fire unite, they produce great power. In the deep breathing produced by tai chi ch'uan and meditation, concentration of the mind is directed toward the lower abdomen, the region of the kidneys. This warming of the lower abdomen helps combine water and fire to make the kidneys healthy.

Benefits for the Skeleton & the Muscles

Tai chi ch'uan, through gentle internal and external movements, prevents sickness, strengthens the internal organs, and makes the mind peaceful. It is highly effective for muscle, skeletal, and joint conditions, too.

Recently, medical doctors have begun to advise patients with arthritis to move slowly and gently. If they move too quickly, they will worsen their condition. If they do not move at all, the arthritic condition will become worse, and they may lose active use of their joints and ligaments. Tai chi ch'uan would appear to be an ideal exercise for such patients.

Tai chi ch'uan movements should be balanced and centered. Age-old books on tai chi ch'uan assert that if your spinal cord is correct and centered, the chi will reach the top of your head. In meditation the chi becomes spirit when it reaches the top of the head. This helps to maintain the body's equilibrium and to prevent backaches and injury to the limbs.

Many people suffer from leg injuries. Young people usually hurt their legs because they lose their balance or because they are extremely tense. In older people, the bone marrow is "dry," the bone density lower, the ligaments shortened, and the joints stiff. These conditions lead to many leg and hip injuries. In many people, especially old people, the legs are usually cold. This means that adequate circulation has not reached the feet.

Tai chi ch'uan and meditation direct the chi, which in turn directs blood circulation to the feet. This helps warm the feet, increases the legs' bone marrow and bone density, and prevents exhaustion. The legs of a tai chi ch'uan practitioner should always be warm. In addition, tai chi ch'uan is particularly effective in keeping the body relaxed and balanced, preventing falls.

Benefits for Mental & Emotional Health

Tai chi ch'uan and meditation can also help prevent and cure mental suffering brought on by various emotional conditions.

Grief: People who have lost a close relative, such as a spouse, child, or parent, feel great sadness. This sadness can easily lead to mental or physical illness.

Fear: When a person gets sick, especially from a serious disease, he or she may fear dying. A peaceful mind can help the body heal itself naturally. The best physicians try to console their patients; even when the illness is very serious, they reassure them and urge them not to worry. Psychology often seems to take the place of medicine.

Desire: Many people are interested in achieving high and powerful positions. When someone is suddenly offered a high position or demanding job, he may become overexcited. Once someone has attained a high position, many problems and pressures may keep him from being as resourceful as he might otherwise be. If he should have to leave that position, he may become very sad.

Desire may involve a craving for wealth or love. When people suddenly become rich or when they fall in love, they are happy and excited. But if one should lose his money or the love of some-one he cares for, he may become so devastated that he may lose his health or even his mind.

Tension: Many people in modern society, especially big-city dwellers, feel tension in daily life. Tension can cause and further complicate psychological and physical disorders.

Anger: According to Eastern medicine, anger inflames the body's internal organs. It is damaging mentally and physically. A man once became so angry that he pounded fiercely on top of a desk and, with his own blows, blinded himself.

Avoiding anger can prevent many external and internal injuries and disorders. Tai chi ch'uan and meditation can help us develop calm, peacefulness, relaxation, tolerance, and clarity of mind so that we can control our everyday mental and emotional reactions, such as grief, fear, desire, tension, and anger. It can also help give us the serenity of good health.

Tai Chi Ch'uan & Self-Defense

Some people are drawn to tai chi ch'uan because they want to learn to defend themselves from physical attack. They may have seen or heard about a skilled practitioner of this art effortlessly sending an assailant flying away to crash against a wall or some other object. This kind of magic certainly has its fascination. However, as people are taught the forms, they begin to realize that tai chi ch'uan is based on self-defense movements.

When an attack comes, we must learn to sense the amount and direction of the opponent's force, neutralize it by not presenting a surface for him to push or strike against, and at the same time, strike him or cause him to lose balance.

The emphasis in tai chi ch'uan is on developing the ability to interpret the opponent's attack and, by shifting one's body, cause him to miss his target. Missing the target and expecting resistance where there is none usually results to some degree in a loss of balance. We capitalize on this mistake and the weakness that results by instantly counterattacking. In practice, the counterattack actually develops while the opponent is going off target. If properly done, only a minimum of force is necessary to send the opponent flying a number of feet or meters away.

People who practice tai chi ch'uan learn through experience that the whole body must be utilized. They have the feet planted, or rooted, firmly in the ground and realize the importance of hip and waist flexibility in both neutralizing an attack and returning force to the opponent. As they practice each form and movement of tai chi ch'uan, they notice that every action is coordinated, with all parts of the body simultaneously in play. They understand the need for a low center of gravity and a balanced stance. They realize directly the negative effect tension can have on performance and the positive effect of a relaxed body in performance.

These ways of using the body and relating to the environment are what we hope to instill with tai chi ch'uan. It becomes obvious that experience in tai chi ch'uan helps us to more easily sense and fulfill the requirements of the form.

How useful is tai chi ch'uan as a defensive art? Many who watch the slow movements of tai chi ch'uan fail to see its value as self-defense. Based on their past experience with martial arts, they expect to see an exhibition of techniques performed with great strength and speed. Tai chi ch'uan, however, depends less on strength and speed than do other martial arts. Again, the major emphasis is on fostering the ability to interpret the direction and force of the opponent's attack and to neutralize this attack by moving the body just enough to cause the opponent to miss his target and lose his balance. The very instant of this disequilibrium must be used to counterattack.

In training, sensitivity and flexibility, rather than physical strength or speed, are stressed. Because of the emphasis on acquiring sensitivity in tai chi ch'uan, those who practice it continue to improve over the years. Our ability to refine our sensitivity does not diminish with advancing age. In contrast, the reliance on strength and speed, characteristic of many other martial arts, becomes increasingly more difficult as we grow older.

Let's also look at martial arts realistically. How often have we had to physically defend ourselves from physical attack? We generally do our utmost to avoid trouble and stay clear of violence. However, many of us may have felt physically threatened at one time or another. We would have felt more secure in the knowledge that if a physical attack had actually occurred, we would have been able to cope with it. Achieving some skill in tai chi ch'uan provides this confidence. However, the most important benefit that tai chi ch'uan training can give is the ability to remain calm in the face of a physical threat. The ability to remain cool allows us to determine the action best for the occasion.

If we are attacked physically, we must defend ourselves. However, in civilized society this extreme occurs rarely. If we are sensitive and alert—what tai chi ch'uan training helps us be— we should be able to take timely and appropriate action to avoid a confrontation. Recognizing danger early enough to avoid it or to prepare to neutralize it is the secret to survival. Self-defense is, therefore, much more than a physical ability to overcome assailants.

We must use physical self-defense only when every other possibility has failed.

NEW-STYLE TAI CHI CH'UAN FORMS

The 82 Forms of New-Style Tai Chi Ch'uan

First Sequence (Forms 1–20)

(1) Preparation *(Yu Pei Shih)*
(2) Beginning *(Chi Shin)*
(3) Ward Off, Left *(Tso Peng)*
(4) Ward Off, Right *(Yu Peng)*
(5) Withdraw and Push *(Ju Feng Shih Pi)*
(6) Single Whip *(Tan Pien)*
(7) Brush Left Knee and Twist Step *(Tso Lou Shi Yao Pu)*
(8) Brush Right Knee and Twist Step *(Yu Lou Shi Yao Pu)*
(9) Brush Left Knee and Twist Step *(Tso Lou Shi Yao Pu)*
(10) Chop with Fist *(Pieh Shen Chui)*
(11) Step, Deflect, Intercept, and Punch *(Chin Pu Pan Lan Chui)*
(12) Withdraw and Push *(Ju Feng Shih Pi)*
(13) Crossing Hands *(Shih Tsu Shou)*
(14) Embrace the Tiger and Return to the Mountain *(Pao Hu Kuei Shan)*
(15) Slanting Single Whip *(Hsieh Tan Pien)*
(16) Punch under Elbow *(Chou Ti Chui)*
(17) Step Back and Drive the Monkey Away, Right *(Tao Nien Hou, Yu Shih)*
(18) Step Back and Drive the Monkey Away, Left *(Tao Nien Hou, Tso Shih)*
(19) Step Back and Drive the Monkey Away, Right *(Tao Nien Hou, Yu Shih)*
(20) Diagonal Flying Posture *(Hsieh Fei Shih)*

Second Sequence (Forms 21–40)

(21) Shoulder Stroke *(Kao)*
(22) Brush Left Knee and Twist Step *(Tso Lou Shi Yao Pu)*
(23) Needle at the Bottom of the Sea *(Hai Ti Chen)*
(24) Fan Penetrates the Back *(Shan Tjung Pei)*
(25) Turn Around and Chop *(Ch'uan Shen Pieh Shen Chui)*
(26) Step, Deflect, Intercept, and Punch *(Chin Pu Pan Lan Chui)*
(27) Withdraw and Push *(Ju Feng Shih Pi)*
(28) Step Forward and Ward Off, Right *(Shang Pu Yu Peng)*
(29) Withdraw and Push *(Ju Feng Shih Pi)*
(30) Single Whip *(Tan Pien)*
(31) Waving Hands in Clouds *(Yun Shou)*
(32) Single Whip *(Tan Pien)*
(33) High Pat on Horse *(Kao Tan Ma)*
(34) Strike with Right Foot *(Yu Teng Cho)*
(35) Strike with Left Foot *(Tso Teng Cho)*
(36) Turn Around and Strike with Left Foot *(Ch'uan Shen Teng Cho)*
(37) Step Forward and Punch Downward *(Chin Pu Tsai Chui)*
(38) Turn Around and Chop with Fist *(Ch'uan Shen Pieh Shien Chui)*
(39) Step, Deflect, Intercept, and Punch *(Chin Pu Pan Lan Chui)*
(40) Strike with Right Foot *(Yu Teng Cho)*

Third Sequence (Forms 41–60)

(41) Strike the Tiger *(Ta Hu Shih)*
(42) Strike with Right Foot *(Yu Teng Cho)*
(43) Strike with Both Fists *(Shuang Feng Kuan Er)*
(44) Strike with Left Foot *(Tso Teng Cho)*
(45) Turn Around and Strike with Right Foot *(Ch'uan Shen Teng Cho)*
(46) Chop with Fist *(Pieh Shen Chui)*
(47) Step, Deflect, Intercept, and Punch *(Chin Pu Pan Lan Chui)*
(48) Withdraw and Push *(Ju Feng Shih Pi)*
(49) Crossing Hands *(Shih Tsu Shou)*
(50) Ward Off, Right *(Yu Peng)*
(51) Single Whip *(Tan Pien)*
(52) Fair Lady Weaving at Shuttle I *(Yu Nu Ch'uan Sho)*
(53) Fair Lady Weaving at Shuttle II *(Yu Nu Ch'uan Sho)*
(54) Fair Lady Weaving at Shuttle III *(Yu Nu Ch'uan Sho)*
(55) Fair Lady Weaving at Shuttle IV *(Yu Nu Ch'uan Sho)*
(56) Ward Off, Left *(Tso Peng)*
(57) Ward Off, Right *(Yu Peng)*
(58) Single Whip *(Tan Pien)*
(59) Single Whip Squatting Down *(Tan Pien Hsia Shih)*
(60) Brush Left Knee and Twist Step *(Tso Lou Hsih Yao Pu)*

Fourth Sequence (Forms 61–82)

(61) Needle at the Bottom of the Sea *(Hai Ti Chen)*
(62) Fan Penetrates the Back *(Shan Tjung Pei)*
(63) Turn Around and Chop *(Ch'uan Shen Pieh Shen Chui)*
(64) Step, Deflect, Intercept, and Punch *(Chin Pu Pan Lan Chui)*
(65) Step Forward and Ward Off, Right *(Shang Pu Yu Peng)*
(66) Withdraw and Push *(Ju Feng Shih Pi)*
(67) Single Whip *(Tan Pien)*
(68) High Pat on Horse *(Kao Tan Ma)*
(69) Turn Around and Strike with Right Foot *(Yu Teng Cho)*
(70) Strike with Left Foot *(Tso Teng Cho)*
(71) Step Forward and Punch Downward *(Chin Pu Tsai Chui)*
(72) Step, Deflect, Intercept, and Punch *(Chin Pu Pan Lan Chui)*
(73) Step Forward and Ward Off, Right *(Shang Pu Yu Peng)*
(74) Withdraw and Push *(Ju Feng Shih Pi)*
(75) Single Whip *(Tan Pien)*
(76) Single Whip Squatting Down *(Tan Pien Hsia Shih)*
(77) Turn Around and Strike with Right Foot *(Ch'uan Shen Teng Cho)*
(78) Chop with Fist *(Pieh Shen Chui)*
(79) Step, Deflect, Intercept, and Punch *(Chin Pu Pan Lan Chui)*
(80) Withdraw and Push *(Ju Feng Shih Pi)*
(81) Crossing Hands *(Shih Tsu Shou)*
(82) Closing *(Shou Shi)*

First Sequence
Forms 1–20

(1) Preparation *Yu Pei Shih*

Movement: Shift your weight completely onto the right leg. Raise the left foot and place it sideways about 12 inches (30 cm) to the left, toes pointing directly ahead, and rest your weight on it. At the same time, bend the elbows slightly outward with the palms facing backward. Pivoting on the right heel, raise the right toes and curve them slightly inward so that the right foot is parallel to the left foot. Both feet now point directly ahead. The weight is centered between the two legs, and the distance between the feet should be equal to the distance between the shoulders.

The shoulders should always be slumped and the chest depressed. The tongue should rest against the hard palate and the mouth should be lightly closed. Keep the spine as straight as possible, the lowest vertebrae hanging in a "plumb line" and the head floating as though suspended from above. Your entire body should be completely relaxed. It is only then that the chi can sink to the dantian. (See photo 1.)

Eyes: Look forward.
Breathing: Inhale; then exhale.
Mind: Concentrate on the dantian.
Self-Defense: Store energy (chi) for self-defense.

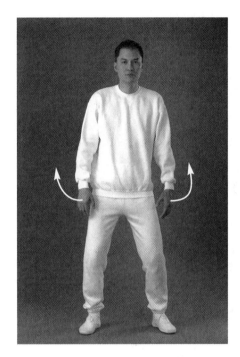

1

Note: Arrows for photos 1–82 (pp. 35–116) indicate the direction of movement.

(2) Beginning *Chi Shin*

Movement 1: Gradually raise the arms forward and upward to shoulder height, with wrists bent, palms facing up, and fingers hanging down. Slowly extend the fingers so that they point forward. (See photo 2A.)

Eyes: Look forward.
Breathing: Inhale.
Mind: Concentrate on the dantian.
Self-Defense: Use all ten fingers to hit an opponent's eyes when he closes in on you.

Movement 2: Bend the elbows slightly and allow the hands to be drawn back toward the upper chest. Lower the elbows slightly as the fingers are raised slightly. Slowly lower your hands (wrists sink as though supported by water, fingers floating upward) until they are below the hip joints with palms facing backward. Bend the elbows slightly outward and let the fingers hang downward. (See photo 2B.)

Eyes: Look forward.
Breathing: Exhale.
Mind: Concentrate on the dantian.
Self-Defense: Put more chi on your hands and palms.

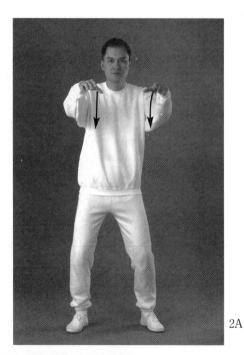

2A

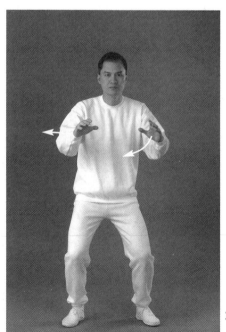

2B

(3) Ward Off, Left *Tso Peng*

Movement 1: Shift your weight to the right foot, and put your right hand at the height of your throat with your palm down and elbow bent. Move your left hand, with the palm up, near the right side of your waist. This posture resembles holding a ball in your hands on the right side of your body. (See photo 3A.)

Eyes: Follow your right hand.
Breathing: Inhale.
Mind: Concentrate on the dantian.
Self-Defense: Put more chi on both hands and palms.

Movement 2: Gradually turn the trunk about 45 degrees to the left so that the left foot is brought to the tip of the toes. Touching first with the heel, place the left foot directly forward, and slowly shift the weight onto it while turning the upper torso to the left. At the same time, raise the left arm with the elbow slightly down. Lower the right arm while pivoting on the heel, turning the right foot inward. Shift 70 percent of your weight to the left foot. At the same time, continue to raise the left arm until the palm faces your chest, and continue to lower the right arm until the hand, with palm down, rests beside the right hip joint. (See photo 3B.)

Eyes: Follow left arm, forearm, and hand.
Breathing: Exhale.
Mind: Direct energy from the dantian to your left arm and hand.
Self-Defense: Use your left arm, forearm, and hand to protect yourself against an opponent's attack on your left side. At the same time, use your right hand to block your right side in case an opponent tries to kick you on that side.

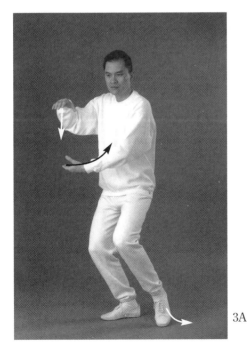

3A

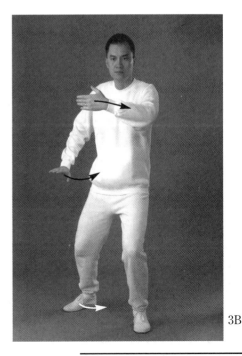

3B

(4) Ward Off, Right *Yu Peng*

Movement 1: Shift all your weight to the left foot. Put your left hand, with palm down, at the height of your throat, keeping the elbow bent. Move your right hand near the right side of your waist with the palm up. This posture resembles holding a ball in your hands on the left side of your body. (See photo 4A.)

Eyes: Follow your left hand.
Breathing: Inhale.
Mind: Concentrate on the dantian.
Self-Defense: Put more chi on both hands and palms.

Movement 2: Gradually turn the trunk about 45 degrees to the right so that you stand on tiptoe with your right foot. Touching first with the heel, place the right foot directly to the right side, and slowly shift your weight onto it while turning the upper torso to the right. At the same time, raise the right arm with the elbow slightly down. Lower the left arm while pivoting on the heel, turning the left foot inward. Shift 70 percent of your weight to the right foot while continuing to raise the right arm until the palm faces your chest. Continue to lower the left arm until the hand rests beside the left hip joint, palm down. (See photo 4B.)

Eyes: Follow right arm, forearm, and hand.
Breathing: Exhale.
Mind: Direct energy from the dantian to your right arm and hand.
Self-Defense: Use your right arm, forearm, and hand to protect yourself against an opponent's attack on your right side. At the same time, use your left hand to block your left side in case an opponent tries to kick you on that side.

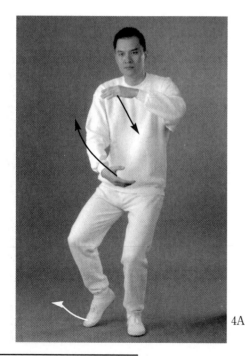

4A

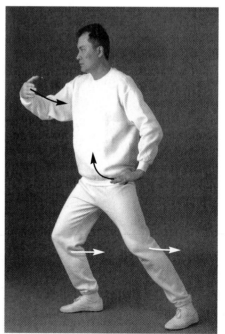

4B

(5) Withdraw and Push *Ju Feng Shih Pi*

Movement 1: Turn both palms down as the left hand passes over the right wrist, moves forward then left, and stops level with the right hand. Separate the hands a shoulder's width apart, and sit back as you shift your weight to the slightly bent right leg. Draw both hands back to the front of the abdomen, palms facing down and slightly to the front. (See photo 5A.)

Eyes: Look forward.
Breathing: Inhale.
Mind: Concentrate on the dantian.
Self-Defense: Use both arms, hands, and palms to grasp your opponent's shoulders toward you, and pull down.

Movement 2: Slowly transfer your weight to the left leg while pushing your hands forward and obliquely up, palms facing forward, until your wrists are shoulder high. At the same time, bend the left knee into a bow step. (See photo 5B.)

Eyes: Follow both hands.
Breathing: Exhale.
Mind: Visualize energy coming from the dantian through both arms to both hands.
Self-Defense: Use both hands and palms to push your opponent's chest away.

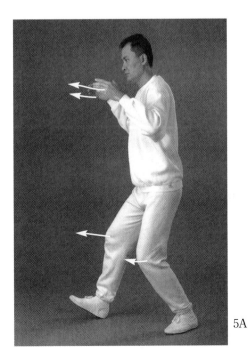
5A

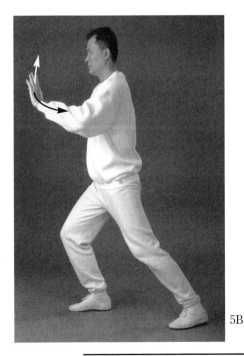
5B

(6) Single Whip (*Tan Pien*)

Movement 1: Shift your weight gradually to the left foot. Turn your torso to the left 180 degrees, and at the same time swivel on the right heel, curving the toes inward as far as possible. As the weight is shifted back to the right leg, allow the body to turn to the right and, as the elbow bends, withdraw the right arm. Allow the fingers to point downward, and close the fingertips together, thus forming a "hook" near the right armpit. Bring the left hand to rest, palm up, near the right breast. (See photo 6A.)

Eyes: Follow your right hand.
Breathing: Inhale.
Mind: Concentrate on the dantian.
Self-Defense: Use your right hand to protect yourself when an opponent closes in on your right side.

Movement 2: As the torso turns toward the left, take a wide step to the left with the left foot. First set the heel down, then the toes, which point left. Shift your weight to the left leg. The left heel should not be directly in front of the right heel but on as wide a diagonal position as you can comfortably manage. Gradually shift the body weight to your left leg, bending the leg at the knee. At the same time, turn the left palm outward with arm slightly bent. (See photo 6B.)

Eyes: Follow your left hand.
Breathing: Exhale.
Mind: Visualize energy coming from the dantian through your left arm to your left hand.
Self-Defense: Use your left hand to attack an opponent on your left side.

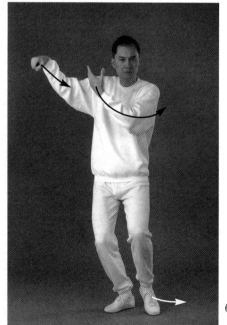

6A

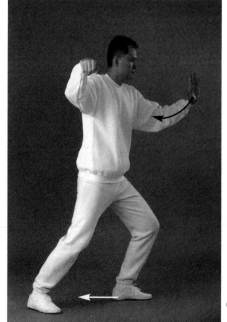

6B

(7) Brush Left Knee and Twist Step *Tso Lou Shi Yao Pu*

Movement 1: The right hand circles downward, backward, and upward, returning to the right side of your head. At the same time, the left hand circles clockwise, backward, upward, and forward to the right ear. This palm should face outward and be slightly down; the elbow should be bent. At the same time, shift your body weight to your right foot. (See photo 7A.)

Eyes: Look forward.
Breathing: Inhale.
Mind: Concentrate on the dantian.
Self-Defense: Use both your right hand and arm and your left hand and arm to protect yourself from a frontal attack.

Movement 2: Turn your torso slightly to the left, and take a big step forward with the left foot, your heel touching the ground first. Brush the left knee with the left hand, palm down, bringing it to rest beside the left thigh. Begin shifting your body weight to the left foot, and curve the right foot slightly inward, turning on the heel. Push your right hand forward, the elbow slightly bent. (See photo 7B.)

Eyes: Follow your right hand.
Breathing: Exhale.
Mind: Visualize energy coming from the dantian through your right arm to your right hand.
Self-Defense: Use your left hand to protect your left knee from an opponent's kick. Use your right hand to attack an opponent in front of you.

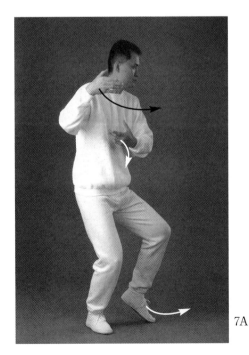

7A

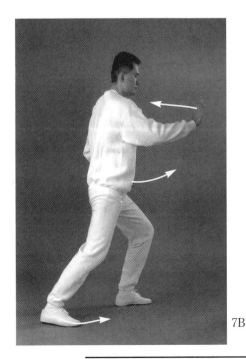

7B

(8) Brush Right Knee and Twist Step *Yu Lou Shi Yao Pu*

Movement 1: The left hand circles downward, backward, and upward, returning to the left side of your head. At the same time, the right hand circles clockwise, backward, upward, and forward to the left ear. This palm should face outward and be slightly inclined down; keep your elbow bent. At the same time, shift your body weight to the left foot. (See photo 8A.)

Eyes: Look forward.
Breathing: Inhale.
Mind: Concentrate on the dantian.
Self-Defense: Use both your left hand and arm and your right hand and arm to protect yourself from a frontal attack.

Movement 2: Turn the torso slightly to the right, and take a big step forward with the right foot, your heel touching the ground first. Brush the right knee with the right hand, palm down, bringing it to rest beside the right thigh. Begin shifting your body weight to the right foot, and curve the left foot slightly inward, turning on the heel. Push your left hand forward, with the elbow slightly bent. (See photo 8B.)

Eyes: Follow your right hand.
Breathing: Exhale.
Mind: Visualize energy coming from the dantian through your left arm to your left hand.
Self-Defense: Use your right hand to protect your right knee from an opponent's kick, and use your left hand to attack an opponent in front of you.

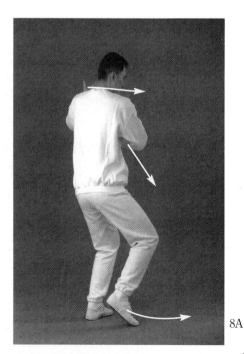

8A

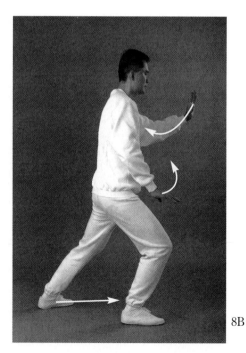

8B

(9) Brush Left Knee and Twist Step *Tso Lou Shi Yao Pu*

Movement 1: The right hand circles downward, backward, and upward, returning to the right side of your head. At the same time, the left hand circles clockwise, backward, upward, and forward to the right ear. This palm should face outward and be slightly inclined downward with your elbow bent. At the same time, shift your body weight to your right foot. (See photo 9A.)

Eyes: Look forward.
Breathing: Inhale.
Mind: Concentrate on the dantian.
Self-Defense: Use your right hand and arm and your left hand and arm to protect yourself from a frontal attack.

Movement 2: Turn the torso slightly to the left, and take a big step forward with the left foot, your heel touching the ground first. Brush the left knee with the left hand, palm down, bringing it to rest beside the left thigh. Begin shifting your body weight to the left foot, and curve the right foot slightly inward, turning on the heel. Push your right hand forward, with your elbow slightly bent. (See photo 9B.)

Eyes: Follow your right hand.
Breathing: Exhale.
Mind: Visualize energy coming from the dantian through your right arm to your right hand.
Self-Defense: Use your left hand to protect your left knee from an opponent's kick, and use your right hand to attack an opponent in front of you.

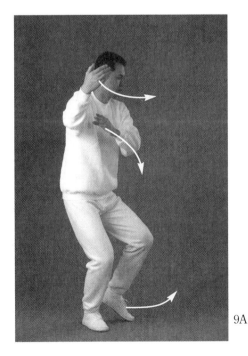

9A

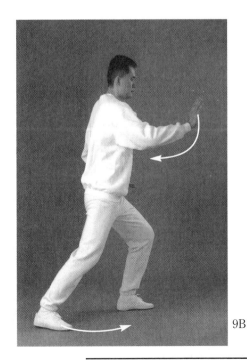

9B

(10) Chop with Fist *Pieh Shen Chui*

Movement 1: Pull your right foot next to your left. At the same time, make a fist with your right hand, and move it past the left rib cage with the fist pointing down. Your left palm should face forward. (See photo 10A.)

Eyes: Look forward.
Breathing: Inhale.
Mind: Concentrate on the dantian.
Self-Defense: Put more chi on both hands and the right fist.

Movement 2: Take one big step forward with your right foot, letting the heel touch the floor first. Slowly shift your weight to your right foot. Snap your fist forward and out, fully extending the arm. (See photo 10B.)

Eyes: Follow your right fist.
Breathing: Exhale.
Mind: Visualize chi coming from the dantian through your right arm to your right fist.
Self-Defense: Use your right fist to attack an opponent in front of you.

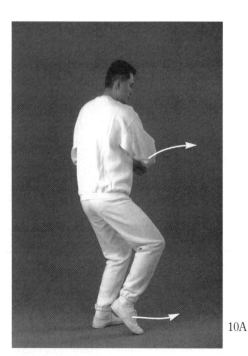

10A

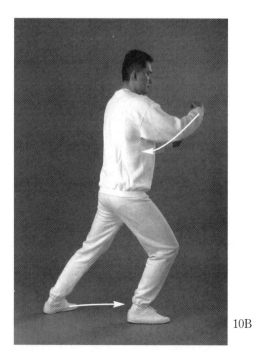

10B

(11) Step, Deflect, Intercept, and Punch *Chin Pu Pan Lan Chui*

Movement 1: Move your right fist in an arc back to your right waist. Begin to bring your left hand up. At the same time, slowly shift your weight to your right foot and take one big step forward with your left foot. Push your left arm forward, your palm facing downward, and your fingertips pointing upward with elbow slightly bent. (See photo 11A.)

Eyes: Follow your left hand.
Breathing: Inhale.
Mind: Concentrate on the dantian.
Self-Defense: Use your left arm and hand to protect your chest.

Movement 2: Shift your weight to your left foot, bending the knee, and punch your right fist forward at chest height. The bottom of your fist should face inward. At the same time, pull your left hand back next to your right forearm, near the elbow. (See photo 11B.)

Eyes: Follow both your arms and hands.
Breathing: Exhale.
Mind: Visualize energy coming from the dantian through both arms to both hands, then to your right fist and left palm.
Self-Defense: Use your right fist to attack an opponent in front of you and your left arm and hand to protect your chest.

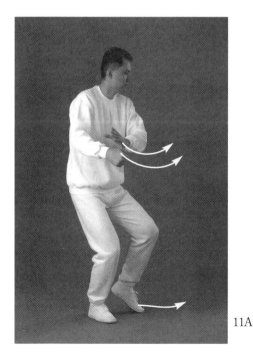

11A

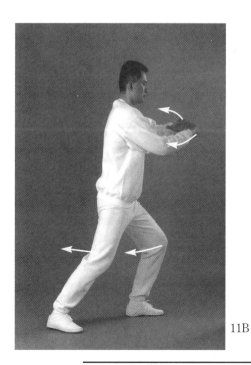

11B

(12) Withdraw and Push *Ju Feng Shih Pi*

Movement 1: Turn both palms down as the left hand passes over the right wrist and moves forward and then left, ending level with the right hand. Separate hands a shoulder's width apart, and "sit" back as you shift your weight to the slightly bent right leg. Draw both hands back to the front of the abdomen, palms facing slightly downward to the front. (See photo 12A.)

Eyes: Look forward.
Breathing: Inhale.
Mind: Concentrate on the dantian.
Self-Defense: Use both arms and hands to grasp your opponent's shoulders and pull them toward you and down.

Movement 2: Slowly transfer your weight to the left leg while pushing your hands forward and obliquely up, palms facing forward, until your wrists are shoulder high. At the same time, bend the left knee into a bow step. (See photo 12B.)

Eyes: Follow both hands.
Breathing: Exhale.
Mind: Visualize energy coming from the dantian through both arms to both hands.
Self-Defense: Use both hands and palms to push your opponent's chest away.

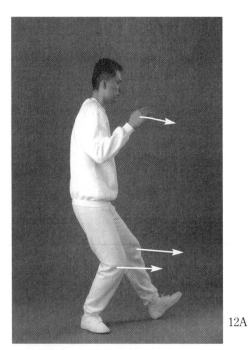

12A

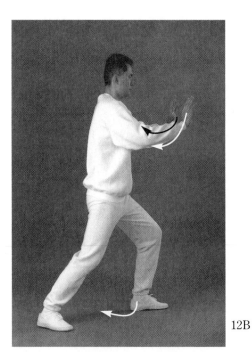

12B

(13) Crossing Hands *Shih Tsu Shou*

Movement: Shift your weight to the right leg, and turn your body to the right with your left heel touching the ground. Bend your right knee and "sit" back. Following the turn of the body, move both hands to your sides in a circular movement at shoulder level, palms facing forward and elbows slightly bent. Slowly shift your weight to the left leg, and turn the toes of your right foot inward. Then bring your right foot toward the left so that both feet are parallel and a shoulder's width apart.

Gradually straighten the legs. At the same time, move both hands down and cross them in front of your abdomen. Raise crossed hands to chest level with your wrists at shoulder level, your right hand on the outside, and your palms facing inward. (See photo 13.)

Eyes: Look forward.
Breathing: Inhale.
Mind: Concentrate on the dantian.
Self-Defense: Use both arms and hands to protect your chest.

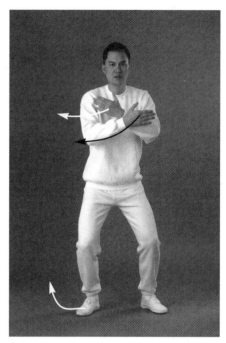

13

(14) Embrace the Tiger and Return to the Mountain *Pao Hu Kuei Shan*

Movement: Turn your body to the right, move a step to your right side, and shift all your weight to the right foot. Move your right hand to the right and backward, and place it beside your right thigh with palm down. The left hand makes a clockwise circle downward, backward, and upward. It stops past the left ear with palm forward and elbow bent. Then push out. Turn your left foot slightly inward. (See photo 14.)

Eyes: Follow your left arm and hand.
Breathing: Exhale.
Mind: Visualize energy coming from the dantian to your left arm and hand.
Self-Defense: Use your right hand to protect yourself against an attack from your right side. Use your left arm and hand to attack an opponent.

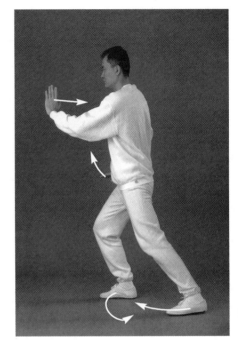

14

(15) Slanting Single Whip *Hsieh Tan Pien*

Movement 1: Shift your weight gradually to the left foot. Turn your torso to the left 180 degrees and at the same time swivel on the right heel, curving the toes inward as far as possible. As you shift your weight back to the right leg, allow the body to turn to the right and, as the elbow bends, withdraw the right arm. Allow the fingers to point downward, and close the fingertips together, forming a "hook" near the right armpit. Bring the left hand to rest, palm up, near the right breast. (See photo 15A.)

Eyes: Follow your right hand.
Breathing: Inhale.
Mind: Concentrate on your dantian.
Self-Defense: Use your right hand to protect yourself when an opponent closes in on your right side.

Movement 2: As the torso turns toward the left, take a wide step to the left with the left foot. First set the heel down, then the toes, which point left. Shift your weight to the left leg. The left heel should not be directly in front of the right heel but on as wide a diagonal position as you can comfortably manage. Gradually shift the body weight to your left leg, bending the leg at the knee. At the same time, turn the left palm outward with arm slightly bent. (See photo 15B.)

Eyes: Follow your left hand.
Breathing: Exhale.
Mind: Visualize energy coming from the dantian through your left arm to your left hand.
Self-Defense: Use your left hand to attack an opponent on your left side.

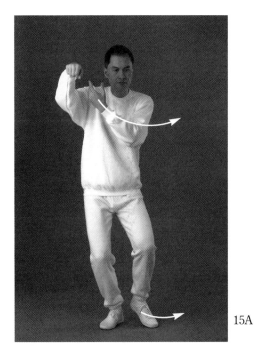

15A

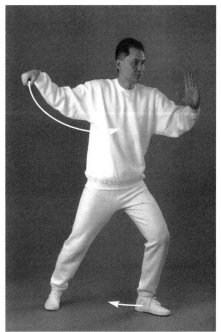

15B

(16) Punch under Elbow *Chou Ti Chui*

Movement: Move your right foot a step, bringing it close to your left foot. Shift your weight back to your right leg with your left heel touching the ground. Then turn your upper torso farther to the left while extending your left arm in front your chest. Hold your right fist and move it under the left elbow. (See photo 16.)

Eyes: Follow your left hand.
Breathing: Inhale first; then exhale.
Mind: First concentrate on the dantian; then visualize energy coming from the dantian through both arms to the left hand and the right fist.
Self-Defense: Use both arms, the left hand, and the right fist to protect yourself from an attack in front of you.

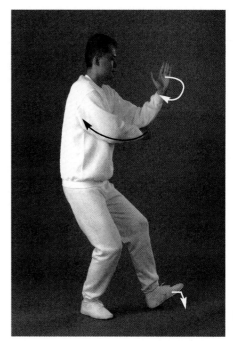

16

(17) Step Back and Drive the Monkey Away, Right *Tao Nien Hou, Yu Shih*

Movement 1: Turn your body right, and open up your palm. Circle your right hand counterclockwise, downward, backward, and upward, and extend it toward the back at shoulder height. At the same time, turn your left hand palm up, and extend it to the front at shoulder height. (See photo 17A.)

Eyes: Follow your right hand.
Breathing: Inhale.
Mind: Concentrate on the dantian.
Self-Defense: Use your left hand and arm to protect yourself from the left and front side, and use your right hand and arm to protect yourself from the right and back side.

Movement 2: Turn your body right, and continue to make a circle with your right hand by bringing it forward and placing it beside your right ear with the palm forward and inclined slightly downward. Then turn your left palm upward, draw it back and downward, and put it beside your left thigh. Draw your right hand downward, with your elbow bent, in front of your chest, your fingers pointing slightly upward. At the same time, step back with your left foot with toes pointing directly in front, and shift your weight to it, curving your toes slightly inward. When most of your weight has been gradually shifted to your left foot, push your right hand forward with the elbow slightly bent and palm outward. (See photo 17B.)

Eyes: Follow your right hand.
Breathing: Exhale.
Mind: Visualize energy coming from the dantian through your right arm to your right hand.
Self-Defense: Use your right hand to attack an opponent in front of you.

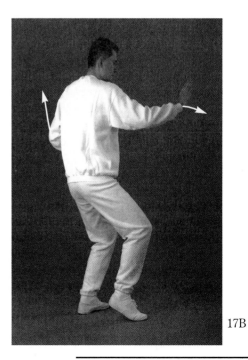

17A

17B

Movement 1: Turn your body left, and open up your palm. Circle your left hand counterclockwise, downward, backward, and upward, and extend it toward the back at shoulder height. At the same time, turn your right hand palm up, and extend it to the front at shoulder height. (See photo 18A.)

Eyes: Follow your left hand.
Breathing: Inhale.
Mind: Concentrate on the dantian.
Self-Defense: Use your right hand and arm to protect yourself from the right and front side, and use your left hand and arm to protect yourself from the left and back side.

Movement 2: Turn your body left, and continue to make a circle with your left hand by bringing it forward and placing it beside your left ear with the palm forward and slightly downward. Then turn your right palm upward, draw it back and downward, and put it beside your right thigh. Draw your left hand downward, with your elbow bent, in front of your chest, your fingers pointing slightly upward. At the same time, step back with your right foot with toes pointing directly in front, and shift your weight to it, curving your toes slightly inward. When most of your weight has been gradually shifted to your right foot, push your left hand forward with the elbow slightly bent and palm outward. (See photo 18B.)

Eyes: Follow your left hand.
Breathing: Exhale.
Mind: Visualize energy coming from the dantian through your left arm to your left hand.
Self-Defense: Use your left hand to attack an opponent in front of you.

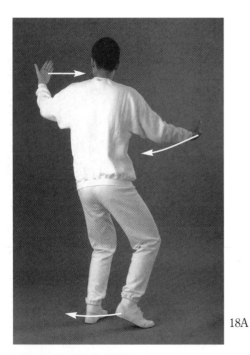

18A

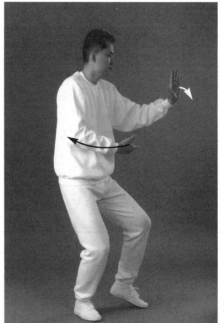

18B

(19) Step Back and Drive the Monkey Away, Right *Tao Nien Hou, Yu Shih*

Movement 1: Turn your body right, and open up your palm. Circle your right hand counterclockwise, downward, backward, and upward, and extend it toward the back at shoulder height. At the same time, turn your left hand palm up, and extend it to the front at shoulder height. (See photo 19A.)

Eyes: Follow your right hand.
Breathing: Inhale.
Mind: Concentrate on the dantian.
Self-Defense: Use your left hand and arm to protect yourself from the left and front side, and use your right hand and arm to protect yourself from the right and back side.

Movement 2: Turn your body right, and continue to make a circle with your right hand by bringing it forward and placing it beside your right ear with the palm forward and slightly downward. Then turn your left palm upward, draw it back and downward, and put it beside your left thigh. Draw your right hand downward, your elbow bent, in front of your chest, with your fingers pointing slightly upward. At the same time, step back with your left foot with toes pointing directly in front, and shift your weight to it, curving your toes slightly inward. When most of your weight has been gradually shifted to your left foot, push your right hand forward with the elbow slightly bent and palm outward. (See photo 19B.)

Eyes: Follow your right hand.
Breathing: Exhale.
Mind: Visualize energy coming from the dantian through your right arm to your right hand.
Self-Defense: Use your right hand to attack an opponent in front of you.

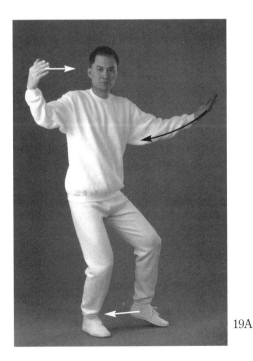

19A

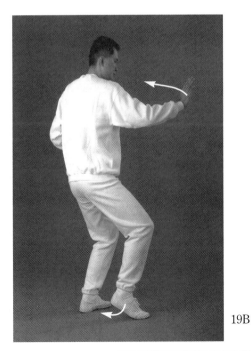

19B

(20) Diagonal Flying Posture *Hsieh Fei Shih*

Movement: Turn your body to the right and take one big step with your right foot to the far right with the heel touching the floor first. Sweep the right arm across to the right and stop at the right side of your head with the turn of the body. The palm is in an upward position. Shift the weight to the right leg and turn the left foot slightly inward. (See photo 20.)

Eyes: Follow your right arm and hand.
Breathing: Inhale.
Mind: Visualize energy coming from the dantian through your right arm to your right hand.
Self-Defense: Use your right arm and hand to protect yourself against attack from the right side.

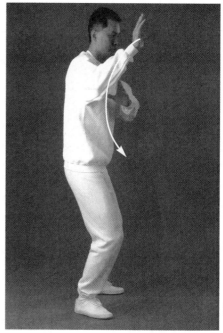

20

Second Sequence
Forms 21–40

(21) Shoulder Stroke *Kao*

Movement: Bring your right foot back and place it down in front of your left heel. At the same time, retract and lower your right hand across your chest, then abdomen, and let it hang by the right side of your waist, palm inward so that the outer edge of the hand is near the front of your right thigh. Lower your left hand and let it hang, palm inward, so that its outer edge is near the outer left thigh. At the same time, shift your weight to your right foot. (See photo 21.)

Eyes: Look forward.
Breathing: Exhale.
Mind: Visualize energy coming from the dantian through your right arm to your right hand.
Self-Defense: Use both hands protect your lower body from an attack in front of you.

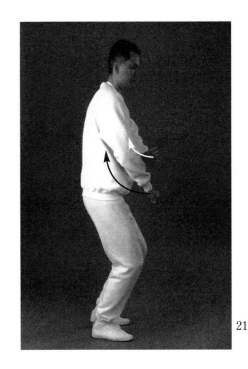

21

(22) Brush Left Knee and Twist Step *Tso Lou Shi Yao Pu*

Movement 1: The right hand circles downward, backward, and upward, returning to the right side of your head. At the same time, the left hand circles clockwise, backward, upward, and forward to the right ear. This palm should face outward and be slightly inclined downward with your elbow bent. At the same time, shift your body weight to your right foot. (See photo 22A.)

Eyes: Look forward.
Breathing: Inhale.
Mind: Concentrate on the dantian.
Self-Defense: Use your right hand and arm and your left hand and arm to protect yourself from a frontal attack.

Movement 2: Turn the torso slightly to the left, and take a big step forward with the left foot, your heel touching the ground first. Brush the left knee with the left hand, palm down, bringing it to rest beside the left thigh. Begin shifting your body weight to the left foot, and curve the right foot slightly inward, turning on the heel. Push your right hand forward, with the elbow slightly bent. (See photo 22B.)

Eyes: Follow your right hand.
Breathing: Exhale.
Mind: Visualize energy coming from the dantian through your right arm to your right hand.
Self-Defense: Use your left hand to protect your left knee from an opponent's kick, and use your right hand to attack an opponent in front of you.

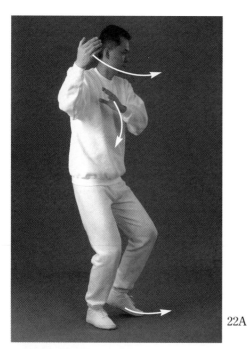

22A

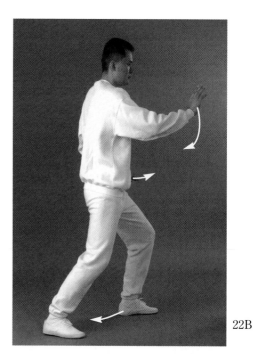

22B

(23) Needle at the Bottom of the Sea *Hai Ti Chen*

Movement: Take half a step forward with your right foot. Shift your weight onto the right leg as your left foot moves forward with the toes coming down on the floor to form a left "empty" step. At the same time, turn your body slightly to the right, lower your right hand in front of your body, then raise it up beside your right ear, and thrust it obliquely downward in front of your body, palm facing left and fingers pointing obliquely downward. Simultaneously, make an arc forward and downward with your left hand until it is beside your left hip with the palm facing downward and fingers pointing forward. (See photo 23.)

Eyes: Follow your right hand.
Breathing: First inhale; then exhale.
Mind: Concentrate on the dantian first; then visualize energy coming from the dantian through your right arm to your right hand.
Self-Defense: Use your left hand to protect your left side, and use your right hand to attack an opponent in front of you.

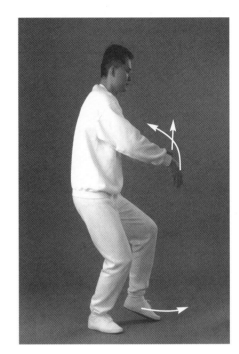

23

(24) Fan Penetrates the Back *Shan Tjung Pei*

Movement: Turn the body slightly to the right. Step forward with your left foot to form a bow step. Shift your weight to your left foot. At the same time, raise your right arm with elbow bent until your hand stops just above your right temple. Turn the palm obliquely upward with the thumb pointing downward. Raise your left hand slightly, and push it forward at nose level, the palm facing forward. (See photo 24.)

Eyes: Follow your left hand.
Breathing: First inhale; then exhale.
Mind: Concentrate on the dantian first, then visualize energy coming from the dantian through both arms to both hands and palms.
Self-Defense: Use your right hand to protect the right side of your head, and use your left hand to attack an opponent in front of you.

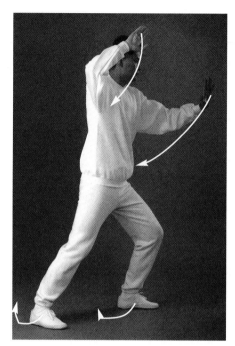

24

(25) Turn Around and Chop *Ch'uan Shen Pieh Shen Chui*

Movement 1: Shift your weight to your right foot, make a right turn 180 degrees, and shift your weight back to your left foot. Pull your right foot next to your left. At the same time, make a fist with your right hand, and move it past the left rib cage with the fist pointing down. Your left palm should face forward. (See photo 25A.)

Eyes: Look forward.
Breathing: Inhale.
Mind: Concentrate on the dantian.
Self-Defense: Put more chi on both hands and the right fist.

Movement 2: Take one big step forward with your right foot, letting the heel touch the floor first. Slowly shift your weight to your right foot. Snap your fist forward and out, fully extending the arm. (See photo 25B.)

Eyes: Follow your right fist.
Breathing: Exhale.
Mind: Visualize chi coming from the dantian through your right arm to your right fist.
Self-Defense: Use your right fist to attack an opponent in front of you.

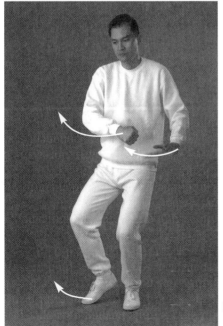

25A

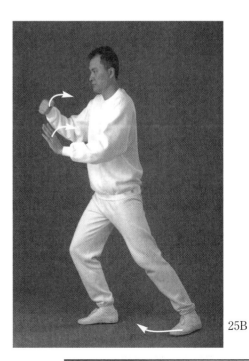

25B

(26) Step, Deflect, Intercept, and Punch *Chin Pu Pan Lan Chui*

Movement 1: In an arc, move your right fist back to the right side of your waist. Begin to bring your left hand up. At the same time, slowly shift your weight to your right foot, and take one big step forward with your left foot. Push your left arm forward, your palm facing downward and your fingertips pointing upward with elbow slightly bent. (See photo 26A.)

Eyes: Follow your left hand.
Breathing: Inhale.
Mind: Concentrate on the dantian.
Self-Defense: Use your left arm and hand to protect your chest.

Movement 2: Shift your weight to your left foot, bending the knee, and punch your right fist forward at chest height. The bottom of your fist should face inward. At the same time, pull your left hand back next to your right forearm, near the elbow. (See photo 26B.)

Eyes: Follow both arms and hands.
Breathing: Exhale.
Mind: Visualize energy coming from the dantian through both arms to both hands, then to right fist and left palm.
Self-Defense: Use your right fist to attack an opponent in front of you and your left arm and hand to protect your chest.

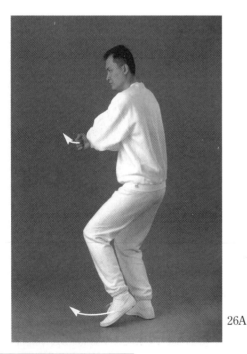

26A

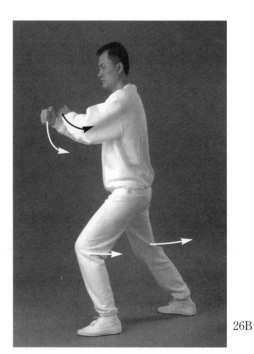

26B

(27) Withdraw and Push *Ju Feng Shih Pi*

Movement 1: Turn both palms down as the left hand passes over the right wrist and moves forward and then left, ending level with the right hand. Separate hands a shoulder's width apart, and "sit" back as you shift your weight to the slightly bent right leg. Draw both hands back to the front of the abdomen, palms facing slightly downward to the front. (See photo 27A.)

Eyes: Look forward.
Breathing: Inhale.
Mind: Concentrate on the dantian.
Self-Defense: Use both arms and hands to grasp your opponent's shoulders toward you and pull down.

Movement 2: Slowly transfer your weight to the left leg while pushing your hands forward and obliquely up, palms facing forward, until your wrists are shoulder high. At the same time, bend the left knee into a bow step. (See photo 27B.)

Eyes: Follow both hands.
Breathing: Exhale.
Mind: Visualize energy coming from the dantian through both arms to both hands.
Self-Defense: Use both hands to push your opponent's chest away.

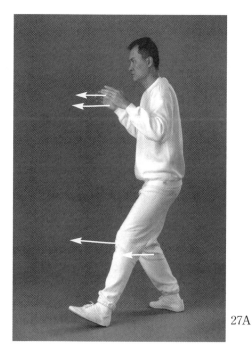

27A

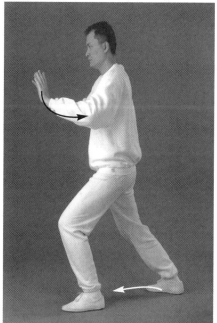

27B

Movement 1: Shift all your weight to the left foot, and put your left hand at the height of your throat with your palm down and elbow bent. Move your right hand near the right side of your waist with the palm up. This posture resembles holding a ball in your hands on the left side of your body. (See photo 28A.)

Eyes: Follow your left hand.
Breathing: Inhale.
Mind: Concentrate on the dantian.
Self-Defense: Put more chi on both hands.

Movement 2: Gradually turn the trunk about 45 degrees to the right so that the right foot is brought to the tip of the toes. Touching first with the heel, place the right foot directly to the right side, and slowly shift the weight onto it while turning the upper torso to the right. At the same time raise the right arm with the elbow slightly down. Continue to raise the right arm until the palm faces your chest, then press your left palm on your right. (See photo 28B.)

Eyes: Follow right arm, forearm, and hand.
Breathing: Exhale.
Mind: Direct energy from the dantian to your right arm and hand.
Self-Defense: Use your right arm, forearm, and hand to protect yourself against an opponent's attack on your right side.

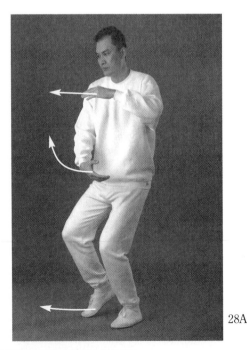

28A

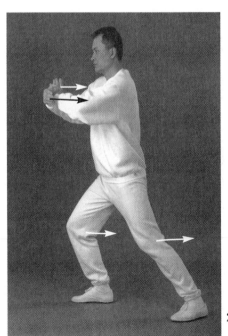

28B

(29) Withdraw and Push *Ju Feng Shih Pi*

Movement 1: Turn both palms down as the left hand passes over the right wrist and moves forward and then left, ending level with the right hand. Separate hands a shoulder's width apart, and "sit" back as you shift your weight to the slightly bent right leg. Draw both hands back to the front of the abdomen, palms facing slightly downward to the front. (See photo 29A.)

Eyes: Look forward.
Breathing: Inhale.
Mind: Concentrate on the dantian.
Self-Defense: Use both arms and hands to grasp your opponent's shoulders toward you and pull down.

Movement 2: Slowly transfer your weight to the left leg while pushing your hands forward and obliquely up, palms facing forward, until your wrists are shoulder high. At the same time, bend the left knee into a bow step. (See photo 29B.)

Eyes: Follow both hands.
Breathing: Exhale.
Mind: Visualize energy coming from the dantian through both arms to both hands.
Self-Defense: Use both hands and palms to push your opponent's chest away.

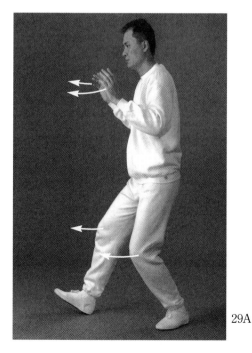

29A

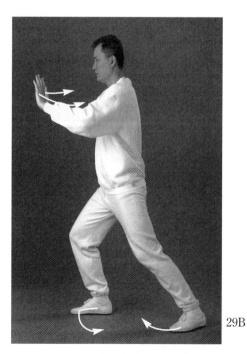

29B

(30) Single Whip *Tan Pien*

Movement 1: Shift your weight gradually to the left foot. Turn your torso to the left 180 degrees and, at the same time, swivel on the right heel, curving the toes inward as far as possible. As the weight is shifted back to the right leg, allow the body to turn to the right, and, as the elbow bends, withdraw the right arm. Allow the fingers to point downward and close them at the fingertips, forming a "hook" near the right armpit. Bring the left hand to rest, palm up, near the right breast. (See photo 30A.)

Eyes: Follow your right hand.
Breathing: Inhale.
Mind: Concentrate on your dantian.
Self-Defense: Use your right hand to protect yourself when an opponent closes in on your right side.

Movement 2: As the torso turns toward the left, take a wide step to the left with the left foot. First set the heel down, then the toes, which point left. Shift your weight to the left leg. The left heel should not be directly in front of the right heel but on as wide a diagonal position as you can comfortably manage. Gradually shift the body weight to your left leg, bending the leg at the knee. At the same time, turn the left palm outward with arm slightly bent. (See photo 30B.)

Eyes: Follow your left hand.
Breathing: Exhale.
Mind: Visualize energy coming from the dantian through your left arm to your left hand.
Self-Defense: Use your left hand to attack an opponent on your left side.

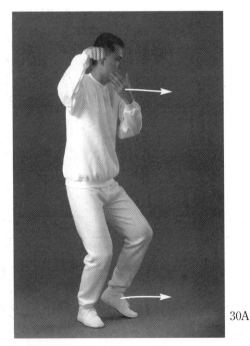

30A

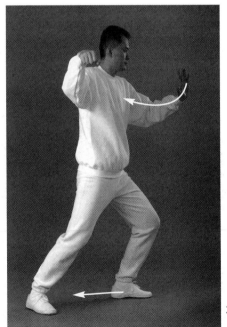

30B

(31) Waving Hands in Clouds *Yun Shou*

Movement 1: First shift your weight to your right foot. Move your left hand down and then up, in an arc, across your abdomen. Start turning your upper body slowly to the right, and turn your left toes inward. Open your right hand and turn it so the palm faces outward and the tips of your fingers point up. (See photo 31A.)

Then bring your left arm up across your abdomen to chest level, and bring your right arm down to your abdomen and up slightly. Turn your upper body to the left. Shift your weight slowly to your left foot. At the same time, continue the arc with your left hand from your face upward to the left, then sideways, down to shoulder level. Simultaneously, move your right arm, in an arc, across your abdomen, and up to your left shoulder. Your right palm should face your shoulder and be turned slightly sideways and up. (See photo 31B.)

Eyes: Follow both hands and palms.
Breathing: Inhale.
Mind: Concentrate on the dantian first; then visualize energy coming from the dantian through both arms to both hands.
Self-Defense: Protect yourself from an attack in front.

Movement 2: Turn your upper body back to your right and shift your weight slowly to your right foot. Make an arc with your right hand upward to your right in front of the face, and bring your left hand up across your abdomen. (See photo 31C.)

Eyes: Follow both hands.
Breathing: Exhale.
Mind: Concentrate on the dantian first; then visualize energy coming from the dantian through both arms to both hands and palms.
Self-Defense: Protect yourself from an attack in front of you.

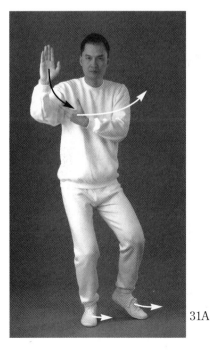

31A

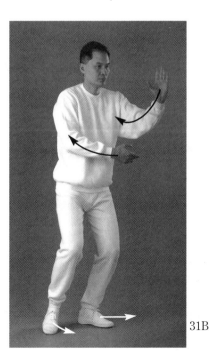

31B

31C

Movement 1: Shift your weight to the right leg. Allow the body to turn to the right and, as the elbow bends, withdraw the right arm. Allow the fingers to point downward and close them at the fingertips, forming a "hook" near the right armpit. Bring the left hand to rest, palm up, near the right breast. (See photo 32A.)

Eyes: Follow your right hand.
Breathing: Inhale.
Mind: Concentrate on your dantian.
Self-Defense: Use your right hand to protect yourself when an opponent closes in on your right side.

Movement 2: As the torso turns toward the left, take a wide step to the left with the left foot. First set the heel down, then the toes, which point left. Shift your weight to the left leg. The left heel should not be directly in front of the right heel but on as wide a diagonal position as you can comfortably manage. Gradually shift the body weight to your left leg, bending the leg at the knee; at the same time, turn the left palm outward with arm slightly bent. (See photo 32B.)

Eyes: Follow your left hand.
Breathing: Exhale.
Mind: Visualize energy coming from the dantian through your left arm to your left hand.
Self-Defense: Use your left hand to attack an opponent on your left side.

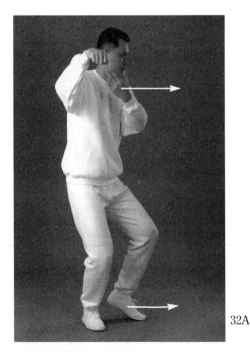

32A

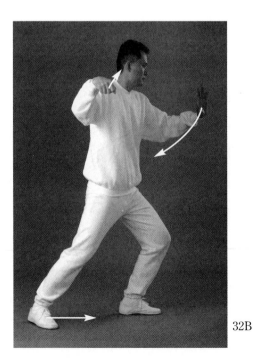

32B

(33) High Pat on Horse *Kao Tan Ma*

Movement 1: Take a half step forward with your right foot as you open your right hand and turn both palms up. Slowly turn your upper body to the right, and shift your weight to your right foot. Raise your right hand to ear level and lift your left foot. (See photo 33A.)

Eyes: Look forward.
Breathing: Inhale.
Mind: Concentrate on the dantian.
Self-Defense: Put more chi on your right hand.

Movement 2: Turn your upper body back to your left and move your left foot forward a step with the heel touching the floor first. Shift your weight to your left foot slowly. Push your right hand forward and cross with your left hand in front of your chest. (See photo 33B.)

Eyes: Follow your right hand.
Breathing: Exhale.
Mind: Visualize energy coming from the dantian through both arms to both hands.
Self-Defense: Use both arms and hands to protect yourself from attack from the front.

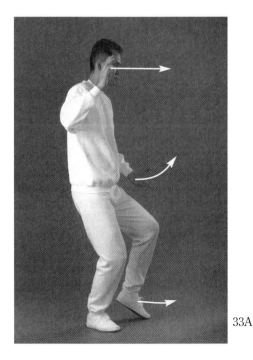

33A

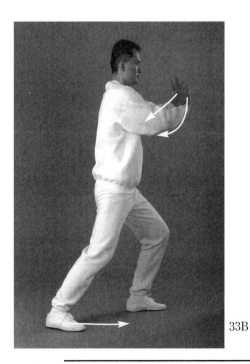

33B

(34) Strike with Right Foot *Yu Teng Cho*

Movement 1: Shift your weight to your left foot. Set your right toes next to your left foot. Continue crossing your hands at chest level. (See photo 34A.)

Eyes: Look forward.
Breathing: Inhale.
Mind: Concentrate on the dantian.
Self-Defense: Put more chi on both hands and right foot.

Movement 2: Slowly turn your body to the right about 20 degrees. Lift your right leg and bend your knee until your thigh is parallel to the floor. At the same time, spread both hands, in an arc, from the crossed position outward. Slowly extend your right foot forward to your right, and continue to extend your arms out at shoulder level. (See photo 34B.)

Eyes: Follow both hands and your right foot.
Breathing: Exhale.
Mind: Visualize energy coming from the dantian through both arms to both hands and through the right leg to the right foot.
Self-Defense: Use both arms and hands as well as the right foot to attack an opponent in front of you.

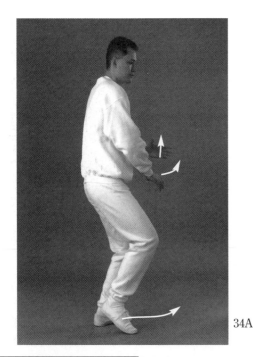

34A

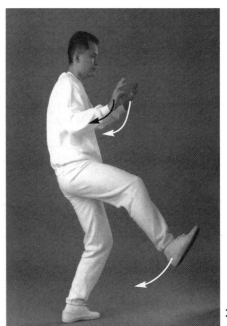

34B

(35) Strike with Left Foot *Tso Teng Cho*

Movement 1: Put your right foot down half a step next to your left foot. Shift your weight to your right foot. Set your left toes next to your right foot. At the same time, withdraw both hands and cross them in front of your chest. (See photo 35A.)

Eyes: Look forward.
Breathing: Inhale.
Mind: Concentrate on the dantian.
Self-Defense: Put more chi on both hands and the left foot.

Movement 2: Slowly turn your body to the left about 20 degrees. Lift your left leg and bend your knee until your thigh is parallel to the floor. At the same time, spread both hands in an arc, from the crossed position outward. Slowly extend your left foot forward to your left, and continue to extend your arms out at shoulder level. (See photo 35B.)

Eyes: Follow both hands and your left foot.
Breathing: Exhale.
Mind: Visualize energy coming from the dantian through both arms to both hands and through the left leg to the left foot.
Self-Defense: Use both arms and hands as well as the left foot to attack an opponent in front of you.

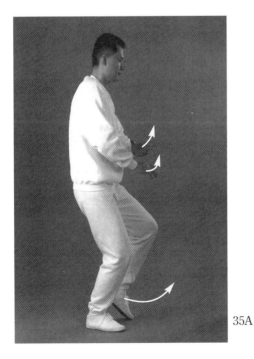

35A

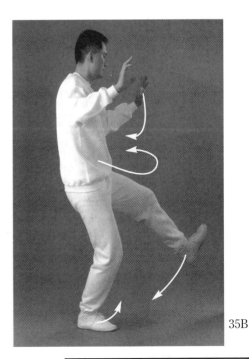

35B

Movement 1: Withdraw both hands and bring them near and cross them in front of your chest. Withdraw your left leg with knee bent and foot suspended in the air next to your right leg. Then swing your body to the left about 180 degrees by turning on your right heel. (See photo 36A.)

Eyes: Look forward.
Breathing: Inhale.
Mind: Concentrate on the dantian.
Self-Defense: Put more chi on both hands and the left foot.

Movement 2: Kick forward with the sole of your left foot with toes upward while chopping forward with both hands at the level of your chest. (See photo 36B.)

Eyes: Follow both hands and your left foot.
Breathing: Exhale.
Mind: Visualize energy coming from the dantian through both arms to both hands and through the left leg to the left foot.
Self-Defense: Use both arms and hands as well as the left foot to attack an opponent in front of you.

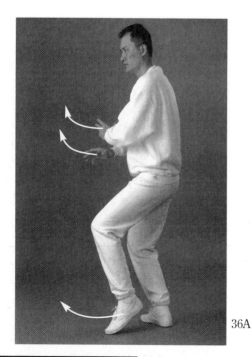

36A

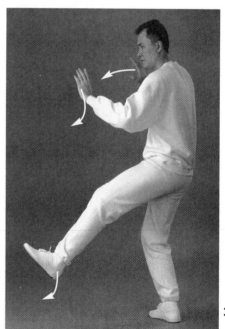

36B

(37) Step Forward and Punch Downward *Chin Pu Tsai Chui*

Movement 1: Put your left foot down a step away from your right foot with the heel touching the ground first.

Eyes: Look forward.
Breathing: Inhale.
Mind: Concentrate on the dantian.
Self-Defense: Put more chi in your right hand.

Movement 2: Shift your weight slightly to your left foot. At the same time, brush your left knee with the left hand, palm down, bringing it to rest beside your left thigh. When 70 percent of your body weight is on the left foot, use the intrinsic energy of your entire body to punch the right fist forward and downward, the elbow slightly bent. (See photo 37.)

Eyes: Follow your right fist.
Breathing: Exhale.
Mind: Visualize energy coming from the dantian through your right arm to your right fist.
Self-Defense: Use your left hand to protect your left knee from an opponent's kick, and use your right fist to attack an opponent in front of you.

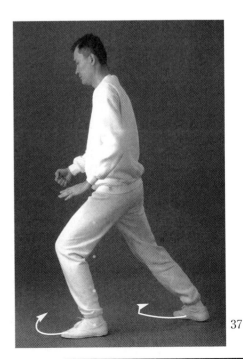

37

(38) Turn Around and Chop with Fist *Ch'uan Shen Pieh Shien Chui*

Movement 1: Shift your weight to your right foot, make a right turn 180 degrees, and shift your weight back to your left foot. Pull your right foot next to your left. At the same time, make a fist with your right hand, and move it past the left rib cage with the fist pointing down. Your left palm should face forward. (See photo 38A.)

Eyes: Look forward.
Breathing: Inhale.
Mind: Concentrate on the dantian.
Self-Defense: Put more chi on both hands and on the right fist.

Movement 2: Take one big step forward with your right foot, letting the heel touch the floor first. Slowly shift your weight to your right foot. Snap your fist forward and out, fully extending the arm. (See photo 38B.)

Eyes: Follow your right fist.
Breathing: Exhale.
Mind: Visualize chi coming from the dantian through your right arm to your right fist.
Self-Defense: Use your right fist to attack an opponent in front of you.

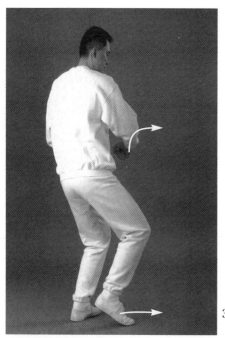

38A

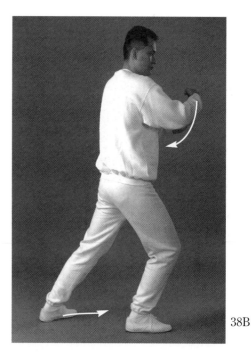

38B

(39) Step, Deflect, Intercept, and Punch *Chin Pu Pan Lan Chui*

Movement 1: In an arc, move your right fist back to the right side of your waist. Begin to bring your left hand up. At the same time, slowly shift your weight to your right foot, and take one big step forward with your left foot. Push your left arm forward, with your palm facing downward and your fingertips pointing upward, elbow slightly bent. (See photo 39A.)

Eyes: Follow your left hand.
Breathing: Inhale.
Mind: Concentrate on the dantian.
Self-Defense: Use your left arm and hand to protect your chest.

Movement 2: Shift your weight to your left foot, bending the knee, and punch your right fist forward at chest height. The bottom of your fist should face inward. At the same time, pull your left hand back next to your right forearm, near the elbow. (See photo 39B.)

Eyes: Follow both arms and hands.
Breathing: Exhale.
Mind: Visualize energy coming from the dantian through both arms to both hands, then to your right fist and left palm.
Self-Defense: Use your right fist to attack an opponent in front of you and your left arm and hand to protect your chest.

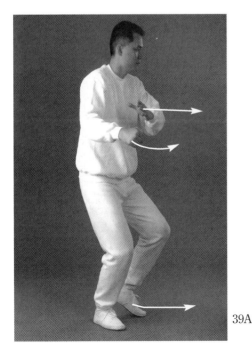
39A

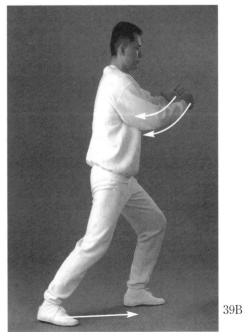
39B

(40) Strike with Right Foot *Yu Teng Cho*

Movement 1: Shift your weight to your left foot. Set your right toes next to your left foot. Continue crossing your hands at chest level. (See photo 40A.)

Eyes: Look forward.
Breathing: Inhale.
Mind: Concentrate on the dantian.
Self-Defense: Put more chi on both hands and the right foot.

Movement 2: Slowly turn your body to the right about 20 degrees. Lift your right leg and bend your knee until your thigh is parallel to the floor. At the same time, spread both hands, in an arc, from their crossed position outward. Slowly extend your right foot forward to your right and continue to extend your arms out at shoulder level. (See photo 40B.)

Eyes: Follow both hands and your right foot.
Breathing: Exhale.
Mind: Visualize energy coming from the dantian through both arms to both hands and through your right leg to your right foot.
Self-Defense: Use both arms and hands as well as the right foot to attack an opponent in front of you.

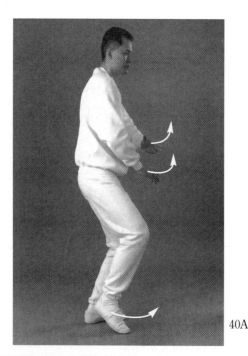

40A

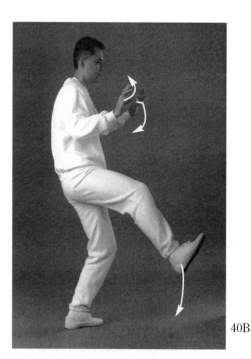

40B

Third Sequence

Forms 41–60

(41) Strike the Tiger *Ta Hu Shih*

Movement 1: Move your right foot down and step forward. Shift your weight to your right foot. At the same time, raise your right arm with elbow bent until your hand stops just above your right temple. Then change your left hand to a fist. Raise your left hand slightly, making a fist, and punch it forward at chest level. (See photo 41A.)

Eyes: Follow your left fist.
Breathing: Inhale.
Mind: Visualize energy coming from the dantian through both arms to both fists.
Self-Defense: Use your left fist to protect your left side, and use your right fist to attack an opponent on your right side.

Movement 2: Make a step to your left with the left foot. Shift your weight to your left foot. At the same time, raise your left arm with elbow bent until your hand stops just above your left temple. Then change your left hand to a fist. Raise your right hand slightly, make a fist, and punch it forward at chest level. (See photo 41B.)

Eyes: Follow your right fist.
Breathing: Exhale.
Mind: Visualize energy coming from the dantian through both arms to both fists.
Self-Defense: Use your left fist to protect your left side, and use your right fist to attack an opponent on your right side.

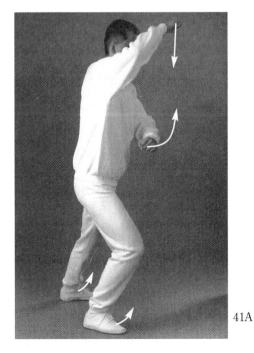

41A

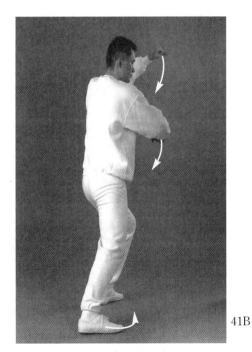

41B

Movement 1: Shift your weight to your left foot. Set your right toes next to your left foot. Continue crossing your hands at the chest level. (See photo 42A.)

Eyes: Look forward.
Breathing: Inhale.
Mind: Concentrate on the dantian.
Self-Defense: Put more chi on both hands and the right foot.

Movement 2: Slowly turn your body to the right about 20 degrees. Lift your right leg and bend your knee until your thigh is parallel to the floor. At the same time, spread your hands in an arc from the cross outward. Slowly extend your right foot forward to your right and continue to extend your arms out at shoulder level. (See photo 42B.)

Eyes: Follow both hands and right foot.
Breathing: Exhale.
Mind: Visualize energy coming from the dantian through both arms to both hands and through the right leg to the right foot.
Self-Defense: Use both arms and hands as well as your right foot to attack an opponent in front of you.

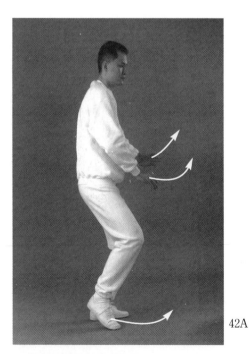

42A

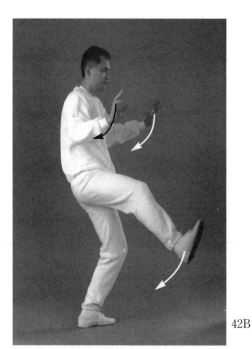

42B

(43) Strike with Both Fists *Shuang Feng Kuan Er*

Movement 1: Lower your right foot until your right heel touches the floor. Lower both hands and, in an arc, start to bring them back up. (See photo 43A.)

Eyes: Look forward.
Breathing: Inhale.
Mind: Concentrate on the dantian.
Self-Defense: Put more chi in both hands.

Movement 2: Take a big step to your right with your right foot. Shift your weight to your right foot and go into the marksman position (see below). Make fists with both hands and bring them toward each other when they reach chest level. Bring both fists in an arc up and forward to ear level, in front of your face. (See photo 43B.)

Eyes: Follow both hands and fists.
Breathing: Exhale.
Mind: Visualize energy coming from the dantian through both arms to both fists.
Self-Defense: Use both fists to attack an opponent in front of you.

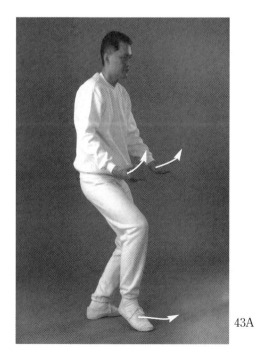

43A

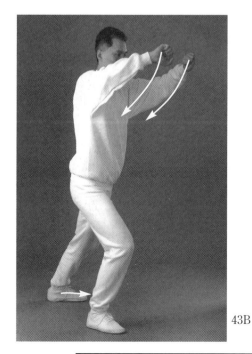

43B

(44) Strike with Left Foot *Tso Teng Cho*

Movement 1: Shift your weight to your right foot. Set your left toes next to your right foot. At the same time, withdraw both hands and cross them in front of your chest. (See photo 44A.)

Eyes: Look forward.
Breathing: Inhale.
Mind: Concentrate on the dantian.
Self-Defense: Put more chi on both hands and on the left foot.

Movement 2: Slowly turn your body to the left about 20 degrees. Lift your left leg and bend your knee until your thigh is parallel to the floor. At the same time, spread both hands in an arc from their crossed position outward. Slowly extend your left foot forward to your left, and continue to extend your arms out at shoulder level. (See photo 44B.)

Eyes: Follow both hands and your left foot.
Breathing: Exhale.
Mind: Visualize energy coming from the dantian through both arms to both hands and through the left leg to the left foot.
Self-Defense: Use both arms and hands, as well as the left foot, to attack an opponent in front of you.

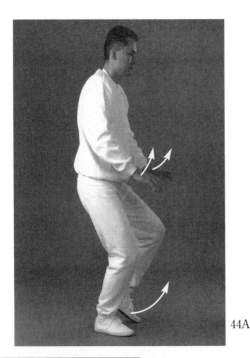

44A

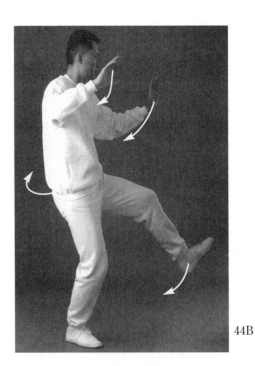

44B

(45) Turn Around and Strike with Right Foot *Ch'uan Shen Teng Cho*

Movement 1: Draw both hands near the body and cross them in front of your chest. Withdraw your left leg with the knee bent and foot suspended in the air next to your right leg. Then swing your body to the right about 360 degrees by turning on your right heel. Put your left foot down half a step next to your right foot. Shift your weight to your left foot. (See photo 45A.)

Eyes: Look forward.
Breathing: Inhale.
Mind: Concentrate on the dantian.
Self-Defense: Put more chi on both hands and on the right foot.

Movement 2: Kick forward with the sole of your right foot with toes upward, while chopping forward with both hands at chest level. (See photo 45B.)

Eyes: Follow both hands and your right foot.
Breathing: Exhale.
Mind: Visualize energy coming from the dantian through both arms to both hands and through the right leg to the right foot.
Self-Defense: Use both arms and hands, as well as the right foot, to attack an opponent in front of you.

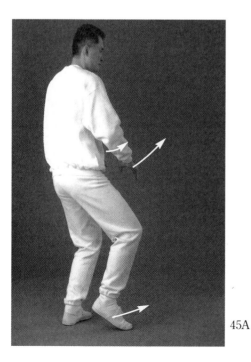

45A

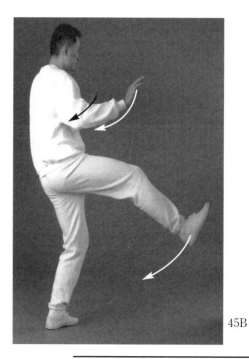

45B

Movement 1: Pull your right foot half a step next to your left foot. At the same time, make a fist with your right hand, and move it past the left rib cage with the fist pointing down. Your left palm should face forward. (See photo 46A.)

Eyes: Look forward.
Breathing: Inhale.
Mind: Concentrate on the dantian.
Self-Defense: Put more chi on both hands and the right fist.

Movement 2: Take one big step forward with your right foot, letting the heel touch the floor first. Slowly shift your weight to your right foot. Snap your fist forward and out, fully extending the arm. (See photo 46B.)

Eyes: Follow your right fist.
Breathing: Exhale.
Mind: Visualize chi coming from the dantian through your right arm to your right fist.
Self-Defense: Use your right fist to attack an opponent in front of you.

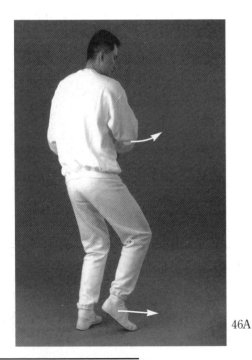

46A

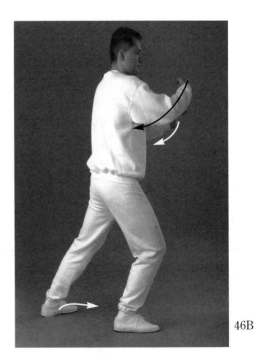

46B

(47) Step, Deflect, Intercept, and Punch *Chin Pu Pan Lan Chui*

Movement 1: Move your right fist in an arc back to the right side of your waist. Begin to bring your left hand up. At the same time, slowly shift your weight to your right foot, and take one big step forward with your left foot. Push your left arm forward, your palm facing downward and your fingertips pointing upward with elbow slightly bent. (See photo 47A.)

Eyes: Follow your left hand.
Breathing: Inhale.
Mind: Concentrate on the dantian.
Self-Defense: Use your left arm and hand to protect your chest.

Movement 2: Shift your weight to your left foot, bending the knee, and punch your right fist forward at chest height. The bottom of your fist should face inward. At the same time, pull your left hand back next to your right forearm, near the elbow. (See photo 47B.)

Eyes: Follow both arms and hands.
Breathing: Exhale.
Mind: Visualize energy coming from the dantian through both arms to both hands, then to the right fist and left palm.
Self-Defense: Use your right fist to attack an opponent in front of you and your left arm and hand to protect your chest.

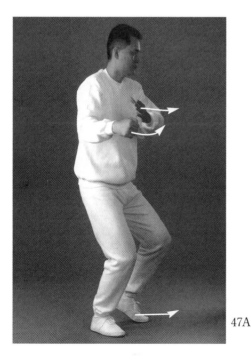 47A

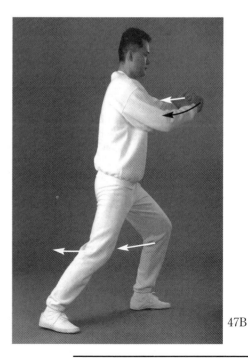 47B

(48) Withdraw and Push *Ju Feng Shih Pi*

Movement 1: Turn both palms down as the left hand passes over the right wrist and moves forward and then left, ending level with the right hand. Separate hands a shoulder's width apart, and "sit" back as you shift your weight to the slightly bent right leg. Draw both hands back to the front of the abdomen, palms facing slightly downward to the front. (See photo 48A.)

Eyes: Look forward.
Breathing: Inhale.
Mind: Concentrate on the dantian.
Self-Defense: Use both arms and hands to grasp your opponent's shoulders toward you and pull down.

Movement 2: Slowly transfer your weight to the left leg while pushing your hands forward and obliquely up, palms facing forward, until your wrists are shoulder high. At the same time, bend the left knee into a bow step. (See photo 48B.)

Eyes: Follow both hands.
Breathing: Exhale.
Mind: Visualize energy coming from the dantian through both arms to both hands.
Self-Defense: Use both hands and palms to push your opponent's chest away.

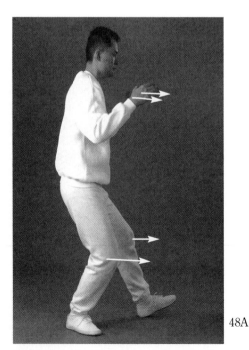

48A

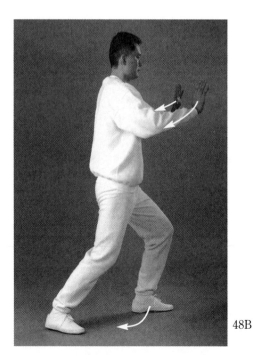

48B

(49) Crossing Hands *Shih Tsu Shou*

Movement: Shift your weight to the right leg, and turn your body to the right with your left heel touching the ground. Bend your right knee and "sit" back. Following the turn of the body, move both hands to your sides in a circular movement at shoulder level, palms facing forward and elbows slightly bent.

Slowly shift your weight to the left leg, and turn the toes of your right foot inward. Then bring your right foot toward the left so that both feet are parallel and a shoulder's width apart. Gradually straighten the legs. At the same time, move both hands down and cross them in front of your abdomen. Raise crossed hands to chest level with your wrists at shoulder level, your right hand on the outside, and your palms facing inward. (See photo 49.)

Eyes: Look forward.
Breathing: Inhale.
Mind: Concentrate on the dantian.
Self-Defense: Use both arms and hands to protect your chest.

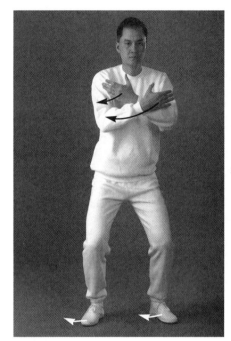

49

(50) Ward Off, Right *Yu Peng*

Movement: Gradually turn the trunk about 45 degrees to the right so that the right foot rises to the tip of the toes. Touching first with the heel, place the right foot directly to the right side, and slowly shift the weight onto it while turning the upper torso to the right. At the same time, raise the right arm with the elbow slightly down. Move your left arm upward and toward your right hand. Shift 70 percent of your weight to the right foot, simultaneously continue to raise the right arm until the palm faces your chest, and press your left palm on your right. (See photo 50.)

Eyes: Follow your upper arms, forearms, and hands.
Breathing: Exhale.
Mind: Direct energy from the dantian to both arms and hands.
Self-Defense: Use upper arms, forearms, and hands to protect yourself against an opponent's attack on your right side.

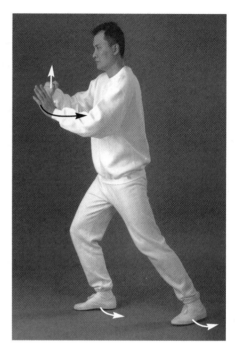

50

(51) Single Whip *Tan Pien*

Movement 1: Shift your weight gradually to the left foot. Turn your torso to the left 180 degrees and at the same time swivel on the right heel, curving the toes inward as far as possible. As you shift your weight back to the right leg, allow the body to turn to the right, and, as the elbow bends, withdraw the right arm. Allow the fingers to point downward and close them at the fingertips, forming a "hook" near the right armpit. Bring the left hand to rest, palm up, near the right breast.

Eyes: Follow your right hand.
Breathing: Inhale.
Mind: Concentrate on your dantian.
Self-Defense: Use your right hand to protect yourself when an opponent closes in on your right side.

Movement 2: As the torso turns toward the left, take a wide step to the left with the left foot. First set the heel down, then the toes, which point left. Shift your weight to the left leg. The left heel should not be directly in front of the right heel but on as wide a diagonal position as you can comfortably manage. Gradually shift the body weight to your left leg, bending the leg at the knee. At the same time, turn the left palm outward with arm slightly bent. (See photo 51.)

Eyes: Follow your left hand.
Breathing: Exhale.
Mind: Visualize energy coming from the dantian through your left arm to your left hand.
Self-Defense: Use your left hand to attack an opponent on your left side.

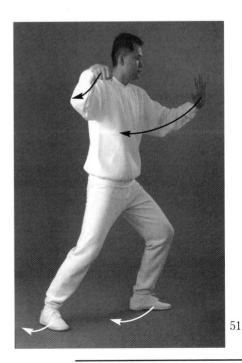

51

(52) Fair Lady Weaving at Shuttle I *Yu Nu Ch'uan Sho*

Movement 1: Turn your torso to the right 180 degrees, and shift your weight to your right foot. Begin to move your hands into the ball-holding position, your right hand on top, in front of your chest to the right. (See photo 52A.)

Eyes: Follow your right hand.
Breathing: Inhale.
Mind: Concentrate on the dantian.
Self-Defense: Use both hands to protect your chest.

Movement 2: Start bringing your right hand down and your left hand up. Turn your body left and take one step forward with your left foot. At the same time, move your left hand in an arc up in front of your chest. Bend your right knee, and shift your weight to your left foot. Continue the arc of your left hand, bringing it up to your face and over to your left temple. Move your right hand up until it points outward and straight. Both palms should face forward. (See photo 52B.)

Eyes: Follow your right hand.
Breathing: Exhale.
Mind: Visualize energy coming from the dantian through your right arm to your right hand.
Self-Defense: Use your left arm and hand to protect your head on the left side, and use your right hand to attack an opponent in front of you.

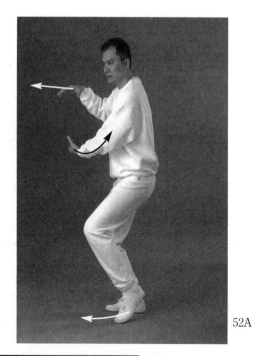

52A

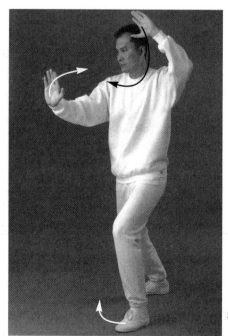

52B

(53) Fair Lady Weaving at Shuttle II *Yu Nu Ch'uan Sho*

Movement 1: Turn your torso to the right 270 degrees and shift your weight to your left foot. Begin to move your hands into the ball-holding position, the left hand on top, in front of your chest to the left. (See photo 53A.)

Eyes: Follow your left hand.
Breathing: Inhale.
Mind: Concentrate on the dantian.
Self-Defense: Use both hands to protect your chest.

Movement 2: Start bringing your left hand down and your right hand up. Turn your body right and take one step forward with your right foot. At the same time, move your right hand in an arc up in front of your chest. Bend your left knee, and shift your weight to your right foot. Continue the arc of your right hand, bringing it up to your face and over to your right temple. Move your left hand up until it points outward and straight. Both palms should face forward. (See photo 53B.)

Eyes: Follow your left hand.
Breathing: Exhale.
Mind: Visualize energy coming from the dantian through your left arm to your left hand.
Self-Defense: Use your right arm and hand to protect your head on the right side, and use your left hand to attack an opponent in front of you.

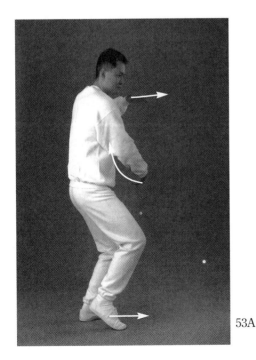

53A

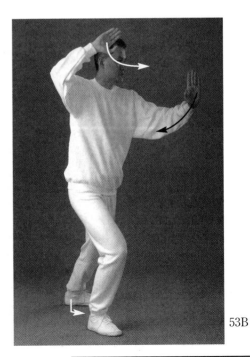

53B

(54) Fair Lady Weaving at Shuttle III *Yu Nu Ch'uan Sho*

Movement 1: Turn your torso to the left 90 degrees, and shift your weight to your right foot. Begin to move your hands into the ball-holding position, right hand on top, in front of your chest, right. (See photo 54A.)

Eyes: Follow your right hand.
Breathing: Inhale.
Mind: Concentrate on the dantian.
Self-Defense: Use both hands to protect your chest.

Movement 2: Start bringing your right hand down and your left hand up. Turn your body left, and take one step forward with your left foot. At the same time, move your left hand in an arc up in front of your chest. Bend your right knee, and shift your weight to your left foot. Continue the arc of your left hand, bringing it up to your face and over to your left temple. Move your right hand up until it points outward and straight. Both palms should face forward. (See photo 54B.)

Eyes: Follow your right hand.
Breathing: Exhale.
Mind: Visualize energy coming from the dantian through your right arm to your right hand.
Self-Defense: Use your left arm and hand to protect your head on the left side, and use your right hand to attack an opponent in front of you.

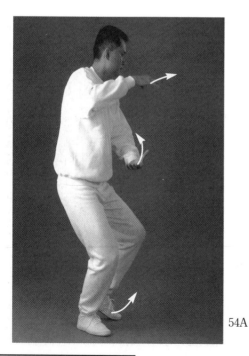

54A

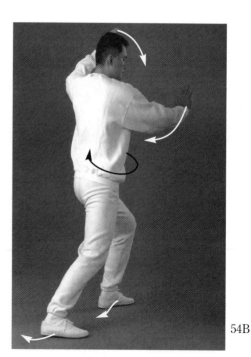

54B

(55) Fair Lady Weaving at Shuttle IV *Yu Nu Ch'uan Sho*

Movement 1: Turn your torso to the right 270 degrees, and shift your weight to your left foot. Begin to move your hands into the ball-holding position, left hand on top, in front of your left chest. (See photo 55A.)

Eyes: Follow your left hand.
Breathing: Inhale.
Mind: Concentrate on the dantian.
Self-Defense: Use both hands to protect your chest.

Movement 2: Start bringing your left hand down and your right hand up. Turn your body right, and take one step forward with your right foot. At the same time, move your right hand in an arc up in front of your chest. Bend your left knee and shift your weight to your right foot. Continue the arc of your right hand, bringing it up to your face and over to your right temple. Move your left hand up until it points outward and straight. Both palms should face forward. (See photo 55B.)

Eyes: Follow your left hand.
Breathing: Exhale.
Mind: Visualize energy coming from the dantian through your left arm to your left hand.
Self-Defense: Use your right arm and hand to protect your head on the right side, and use your left hand to attack an opponent in front of you.

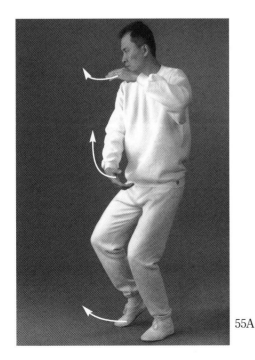

55A

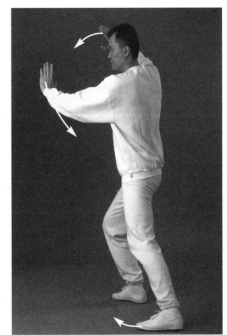

55B

(56) Ward Off, Left *Tso Peng*

Movement 1: Shift your weight to the right foot, and put your right hand at the height of your throat with your palm down and elbow bent. Move your left hand near the right side of your waist with the palm upward. This posture resembles holding a ball in your hands on the right side of your body. (See photo 56A.)

Eyes: Follow your right hand.
Breathing: Inhale.
Mind: Concentrate on the dantian.
Self-Defense: Put more chi on both hands and palms.

Movement 2: Gradually turn the trunk about 60 degrees to the left so that the left foot is brought to the tip of the toes. Touching first with the heel, place the left foot directly forward and slowly shift the weight onto it while turning the upper torso to the left. At the same time, raise the left arm with the elbow slightly down. Move your right hand upward and toward your left hand. Continue to raise the left arm until the palm faces your chest and continue to press your right palm on the left wrist. (See photo 56B.)

Eyes: Follow your upper arms, forearms, and hands.
Breathing: Exhale.
Mind: Direct energy from the dantian to both arms and hands.
Self-Defense: Use your upper arms, forearms, and hands to protect yourself against an opponent's attack on your front side.

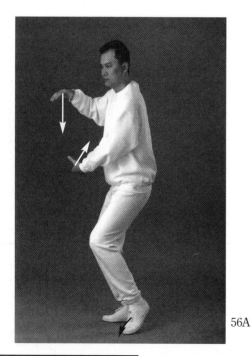

56A

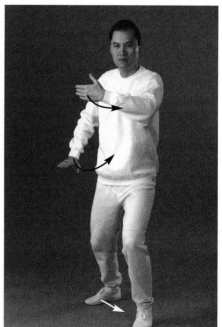

56B

Movement 1: Shift all your weight to the left foot, and put your left hand at the height of your throat with your palm down and elbow bent. Move your right hand near the right side of your waist with the palm upward. This posture resembles holding a ball in your hands on the left side of your body. (See photo 57A.)

Eyes: Follow your left hand.
Breathing: Inhale.
Mind: Concentrate on the dantian.
Self-Defense: Put more chi on both hands and palms.

Movement 2: Gradually turn the trunk about 60 degrees to the right so that the right foot is brought to the tip of the toes. Touching first with the heel, place the right foot directly to the right side, and slowly shift the weight onto it while turning the upper torso to the right. At the same time, raise the right arm with the elbow slightly down. Move your left hand upward and toward your right hand. Continue to raise the right arm until the palm faces your chest, and continue to press your left palm on your right wrist. (See photo 57B.)

Eyes: Follow your upper arms, forearms, and hands.
Breathing: Exhale.
Mind: Direct energy from the dantian to both arms and hands.
Self-Defense: Use your upper arms, forearms, and hands to protect yourself against an opponent's attack on your front side.

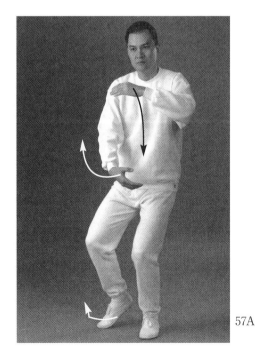

57A

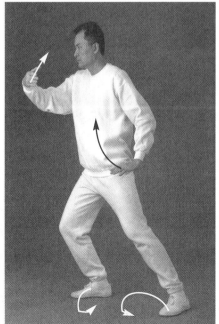

57B

Movement 1: Shift your weight gradually to the left foot. Turn your torso to the left 180 degrees and, at the same time, swivel on the right heel, curving the toes inward as far as possible. As you shift your weight back to the right leg, allow the body to turn to the right and, as the elbow bends, withdraw the right arm. Allow the fingers to point downward and close them at the fingertips, forming a "hook" near the right armpit. Bring the left hand to rest, palm up, near the right breast. (See photo 58A.)

Eyes: Follow your right hand.
Breathing: Inhale.
Mind: Concentrate on the dantian.
Self-Defense: Use your right hand to protect yourself when an opponent closes in on your right side.

Movement 2: As the torso turns toward the left, take a wide step to the left with the left foot. First set the heel down, then the toes, which point left. Shift your weight to the left leg. The left heel should not be directly in front of the right heel but on as wide a diagonal position as you can comfortably manage. Gradually shift the body weight to your left leg, bending the leg at the knee. At the same time, turn the left palm outward with arm slightly bent. (See photo 58B.)

Eyes: Follow your left hand.
Breathing: Exhale.
Mind: Visualize energy coming from the dantian through your left arm to your left hand.
Self-Defense: Use your left hand to attack an opponent on your left side.

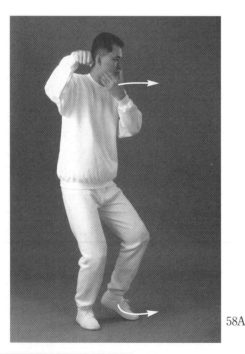

58A

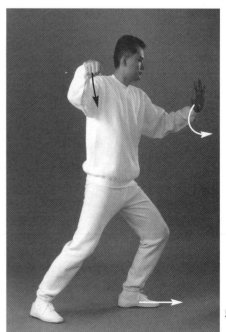

58B

(59) Single Whip Squatting Down *Tan Pien Hsia Shih*

Movement 1: Slowly bend your right knee and extend your left foot to your side, slightly touching the floor. At the same time, let your left hand fall down in an arc across the inside of your left leg. Slowly lower your body as far as your right knee can bend. Do not force yourself too hard; your flexibility will improve over time. Finish the arc with your left hand by bringing it above your outstretched leg, and start to bring it up. Keep your right hand in the hook and start to bring it in an arc down to your hip. (See photo 59A.)

Eyes: Follow your left hand.
Breathing: Inhale.
Mind: Visualize energy coming from the dantian through your left arm to your left hand.
Self-Defense: Use your left arm and hand to protect your lower body.

Movement 2: Turn your left toes outward as far as possible. Use your heel as the axis. Shift your weight to your left foot, and bend your left knee. Extend your right leg and turn your toes inward. Turn your upper body slightly to the left. Raise yourself up with a forward movement as you shift your weight. At the same time, move your right hand in an arc forward and up to shoulder level. (See photo 59B.)

Eyes: Follow your right hand.
Breathing: Exhale.
Mind: Visualize energy coming from the dantian through your right arm to your right hand.
Self-Defense: Use your right arm and hand to protect yourself against an attack in front of you.

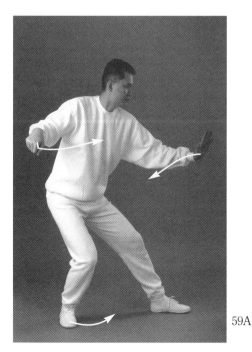

59A

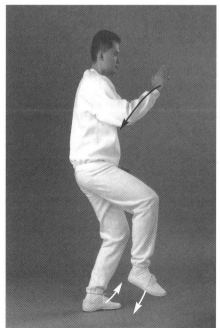

59B

(60) Brush Left Knee and Twist Step *Tso Lou Hsih Yao Pu*

Movement 1: Put your right foot down a half step next to your left foot. Shift your weight to your right foot. Lower your right hand and put it beside your right thigh with the palm down. Raise your left hand forward and up to head level with the elbow bent, fingers pointing up and palm toward your face. At the same time, lift up your left foot with the toes pointing down and the knee bent. (See photo 60A.)

Eyes: Follow your left hand.
Breathing: Inhale.
Mind: Visualize energy coming from the dantian through your left arm to your left hand.
Self-Defense: Use your left arm and hand to protect your face.

Movement 2: Turn the torso slightly to the left, and take a big step forward with the left foot, your heel touching the ground first. Brush the left knee with the left hand, palm down, bringing it to rest beside the left thigh. Begin shifting your body weight to the left foot, and curve the right foot slightly inward, turning on the heel. Push your right hand forward, the elbow slightly bent. (See photo 60B.)

Eyes: Follow your right hand.
Breathing: Exhale.
Mind: Visualize energy coming from the dantian through your right arm to your right hand.
Self-Defense: Use your left hand to protect your left knee from an opponent's kick, and use your right hand to attack an opponent in front of you.

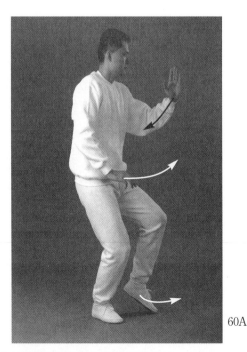

60A

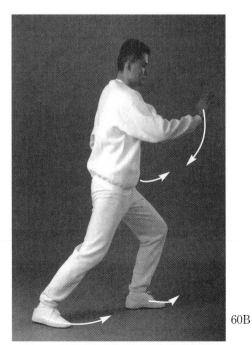

60B

Fourth Sequence
Forms 61–82

(61) Needle at the Bottom of the Sea
Hai Ti Chen

Movement: Take half a step forward with your right foot. Shift your weight onto the right leg as your left foot moves forward with the toes coming down on the floor to form a left "empty" step. At the same time, turn your body slightly to the right, lower your right hand in front of your body, then raise it up beside your right ear, and thrust it obliquely downward in front of your body, palm facing left and fingers pointing obliquely downward. Simultaneously, make an arc forward and downward with your left hand to beside your left hip with the palm facing downward and fingers pointing forward. (See photo 61.)

Eyes: Follow your right hand.
Breathing: First inhale; then exhale.
Mind: Concentrate on the dantian first; then visualize energy coming from the dantian through your right arm to your right hand.
Self-Defense: Use your left hand to protect your left side, and use your right hand to attack an opponent in front of you.

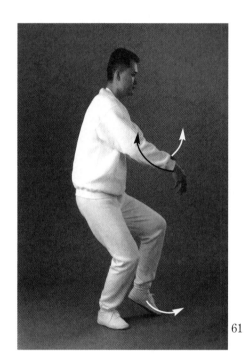

61

(62) Fan Penetrates the Back *Shan Tjung Pei*

Movement: Turn the body slightly to the right. Step forward with your left foot to form a bow step. Shift your weight to your left foot. At the same time, raise your right arm with the elbow bent until your hand stops just above your right temple. Turn the palm obliquely upward with the thumb pointing downward. Raise your left hand slightly, and push it forward at nose level with the palm facing forward. (See photo 62.)

Eyes: Follow your left hand.
Breathing: First inhale; then exhale.
Mind: Concentrate on the dantian first; then visualize energy coming from the dantian through both arms to both hands.
Self-Defense: Use your right hand to protect the right side of your head, and use your left hand to attack an opponent in front of you.

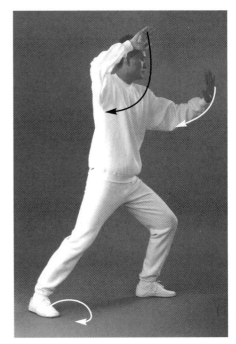

62

(63) Turn Around and Chop *Ch'uan Shen Pieh Shen Chui*

Movement 1: Shift your weight to the right foot, make a right turn 180 degrees, and shift your weight back to your left foot. Pull your right foot next to your left. At the same time, make a fist with your right hand, and move it past the left rib cage with the fist pointing down. Your left palm should face forward. (See photo 63A.)

Eyes: Look forward.
Breathing: Inhale.
Mind: Concentrate on the dantian.
Self-Defense: Put more chi on both hands and the right fist.

Movement 2: Take one big step forward with your right foot, letting the heel touch the floor first. Slowly shift your weight to your right foot. Snap your fist forward and out, fully extending the arm. (See photo 63B.)

Eyes: Follow your right fist.
Breathing: Exhale.
Mind: Visualize chi coming from the dantian through your right arm to your right fist.
Self-Defense: Use your right fist to attack an opponent in front of you.

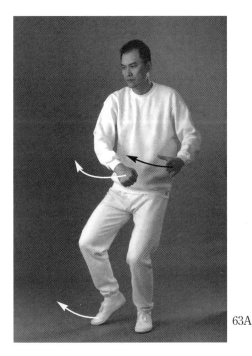

63A

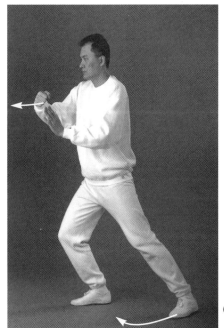

63B

Movement 1: Move your right fist in an arc back to the right side of your waist. Begin to bring your left hand up. At the same time, slowly shift your weight to your right foot, and take one big step forward with your left foot. Push your left arm forward, your palm facing downward, your fingertips pointing upward, and the elbow slightly bent. (See photo 64A.)

Eyes: Follow your left hand.
Breathing: Inhale.
Mind: Concentrate on the dantian.
Self-Defense: Use your left arm and hand to protect your chest.

Movement 2: Shift your weight to your left foot, bending the knee, and punch your right fist forward at chest height. The bottom of your fist should face inward. At the same time, pull your left hand back next to your right forearm, near the elbow. (See photo 64B.)

Eyes: Follow both arms and hands.
Breathing: Exhale.
Mind: Visualize energy coming from the dantian through both arms to both hands, then to the right fist and the left palm.
Self-Defense: Use your right fist to attack an opponent in front of you and your left arm and hand to protect your chest.

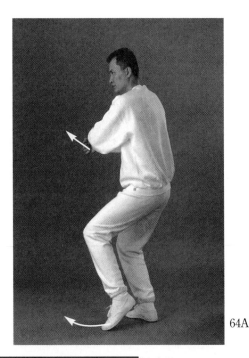

64A

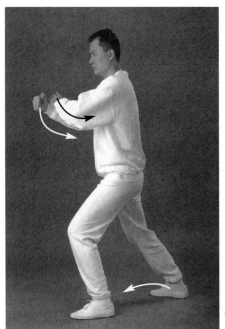

64B

(65) Step Forward and Ward Off, Right *Shang Pu Yu Peng*

Movement 1: Shift all weight to the left foot, and put your left hand at the height of your throat with the palm down and elbow bent. Move your right hand near the right side of your waist with the palm upward. This posture resembles holding a ball in your hands on the left side of your body. (See photo 65A.)

Eyes: Follow your left hand.
Breathing: Inhale.
Mind: Concentrate on the dantian.
Self-Defense: Put more chi on both hands and palms.

Movement 2: Gradually turn the trunk about 60 degrees to the right so that the right foot rises to the tip of the toes. Touching first with the heel, place the right foot directly to the right side, and slowly shift the weight onto it while turning the upper torso to the right. At the same time, raise the right arm with the elbow slightly down. Continue to raise the right arm until the palm faces your chest; then press your left palm on your right wrist. (See photo 65B.)

Eyes: Follow your right upper arm, forearm, and hand.
Breathing: Exhale.
Mind: Direct energy from the dantian to your right arm and hand.
Self-Defense: Use your right upper arm, forearm, and hand to protect yourself against an opponent's attack on your right side.

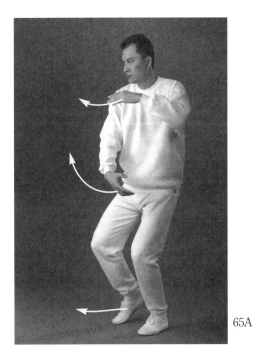

65A

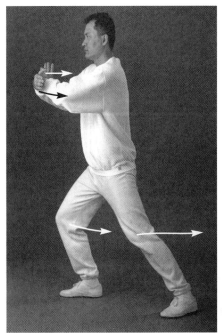

65B

Movement 1: Turn both palms down as the left hand passes over the right wrist and moves forward and then left, ending level with the right hand. Separate hands a shoulder's width apart, and "sit" back (see photo below) as you shift your weight to the slightly bent right leg. Draw both hands back to the front of the abdomen, palms facing slightly downward to the front. (See photo 66A.)

Eyes: Look forward.
Breathing: Inhale.
Mind: Concentrate on the dantian.
Self-Defense: Use your arms and hands to grasp your opponent's shoulders toward you and pull down.

Movement 2: Slowly transfer your weight to the left leg while pushing your hands forward and obliquely up, palms facing forward, until your wrists are shoulder high. At the same time, bend the left knee into a bow step. (See photo 66B.)

Eyes: Follow both hands.
Breathing: Exhale.
Mind: Visualize energy coming from the dantian through both arms to both hands.
Self-Defense: Use both hands and palms to push your opponent's chest away.

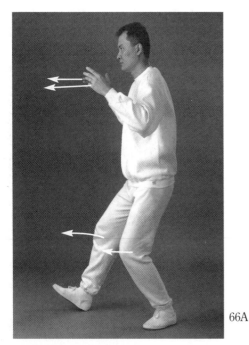

66A

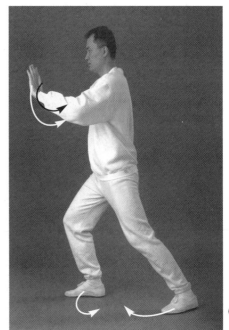

66B

(67) Single Whip *Tan Pien*

Movement 1: Shift your weight gradually to the left foot. Turn your torso to the left 180 degrees and, at the same time, swivel on the right heel, curving the toes inward as far as possible. As you shift the weight back to the right leg, allow the body to turn to the right and, as the elbow bends, withdraw the right arm. Allow the fingers to point downward and close them at the fingertips, forming a "hook" near the right armpit. Bring the left hand to rest, palm up, near the right breast. (See photo 67A.)

Eyes: Follow your right hand.
Breathing: Inhale.
Mind: Concentrate on your dantian.
Self-Defense: Use your right hand to protect yourself when an opponent closes in on your right side.

Movement 2: As the torso turns toward the left, take a wide step to the left with the left foot. First set the heel down, then the toes, which point left. Shift your weight to the left leg. The left heel should not be directly in front of the right heel but on as wide a diagonal position as you can comfortably manage. Gradually shift the body weight to your left leg, bending the leg at the knee. At the same time, turn the left palm outward, with arm slightly bent. (See photo 67B.)

Eyes: Follow your left hand.
Breathing: Exhale.
Mind: Visualize energy coming from the dantian through your left arm to your left hand.
Self-Defense: Use your left hand to attack an opponent on your left side.

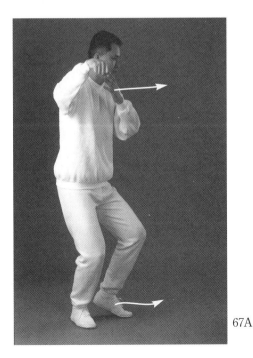

67A

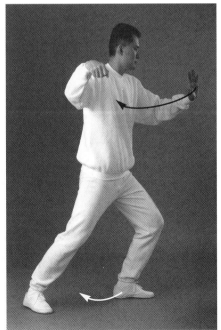

67B

(68) High Pat on Horse *Kao Tan Ma*

Movement 1: Take a half step forward with your right foot as you open your right hand and turn both palms up. Slowly turn your upper body to the right, and shift your weight to your right foot. Raise your right hand to ear level, and lift your left foot. (See photo 68A.)

Eyes: Look forward.
Breathing: Inhale.
Mind: Concentrate on the dantian.
Self-Defense: Put more chi on your right hand.

Movement 2: Turn your upper body back to your left, and move your left foot forward a step with the heel touching the floor first. Shift your weight to your left foot slowly. Push your right hand forward and cross it with your left hand in front of your chest. (See photo 68B.)

Eyes: Follow your right hand.
Breathing: Exhale.
Mind: Visualize energy coming from the dantian through both arms to both hands.
Self-Defense: Use both arms and hands to protect yourself from attack from the front.

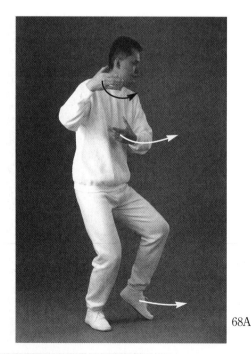

68A

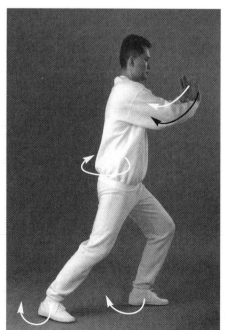

68B

(69) Turn Around and Strike with Right Foot *Yu Teng Cho*

Movement 1: Shift your weight to your right foot, and turn your body to the right 180 degrees. Then shift your weight back to your left foot. Set your right toes next to the left foot. Continue crossing your hands at chest level. (See photo 69A.)

Eyes: Look forward.
Breathing: Inhale.
Mind: Concentrate on the dantian.
Self-Defense: Put more chi on both hands and on the right foot.

Movement 2: Slowly turn your body to the right about 20 degrees. Lift your right leg, and bend your knee until your thigh is parallel to the floor. At the same time, spread both hands in an arc from the crossed position outward. Slowly extend your right foot forward to your right, and continue to extend your arms out at shoulder level. (See photo 69B.)

Eyes: Follow both hands and your right foot.
Breathing: Exhale.
Mind: Visualize energy coming from the dantian through both arms to both hands and through the right leg to the right foot.
Self-Defense: Use both arms and hands as well as your right foot to attack an opponent in front of you.

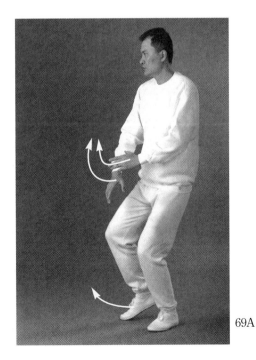

69A

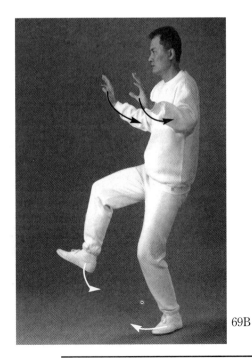

69B

(70) Strike with Left Foot *Tso Teng Cho*

Movement 1: Put your right foot down a half step next to your left foot. Shift your weight to your right foot. Set your left toes next to your right foot. At the same time, withdraw both hands and cross them in front of your chest. (See photo 70A.)

Eyes: Look forward.
Breathing: Inhale.
Mind: Concentrate on the dantian.
Self-Defense: Put more chi on both hands and the on the left foot.

Movement 2: Slowly turn your body to the left about 20 degrees. Lift your left leg, and bend your knee until your thigh is parallel to the floor. At the same time, spread both hands in an arc from their crossed position outward. Slowly extend your left foot forward to your left, and continue to extend your arms out at shoulder level. (See photo 70B.)

Eyes: Follow both hands and your left foot.
Breathing: Exhale.
Mind: Visualize energy coming from the dantian through both arms to both hands and through the left leg to the left foot.
Self-Defense: Use both arms and hands as well as the left foot to attack an opponent in front of you.

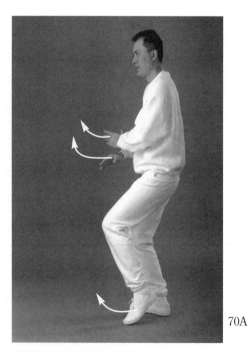

70A

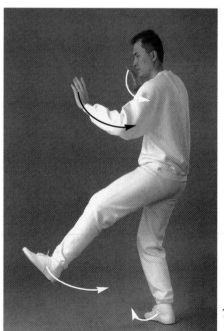

70B

(71) Step Forward and Punch Downward *Chin Pu Tsai Chui*

Movement 1: Put your left foot down a step away from your right foot, the heel touching the ground first. (See photo 71A.)

Eyes: Look forward.
Breathing: Inhale.
Mind: Concentrate on the dantian.
Self-Defense: Put more chi on your right hand.

Movement 2: Shift your weight slightly to your left foot. At the same time, brush your left knee with the left hand, palm down, bringing it to rest beside your left thigh. When 70 percent of your body weight is on the left foot, use the intrinsic energy of your entire body to punch the right fist forward and downward, the elbow slightly bent. (See photo 71B.)

Eyes: Follow your right fist.
Breathing: Exhale.
Mind: Visualize energy coming from the dantian through your right arm to your right fist.
Self-Defense: Use your left hand to protect your left knee from an opponent's kick, and use your right fist to attack an opponent in front of you.

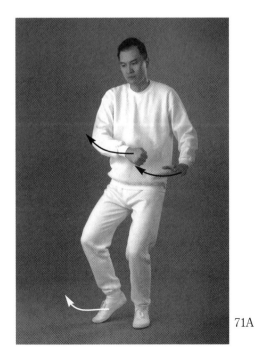

71A

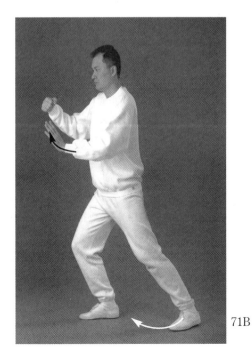

71B

(72) Step, Deflect, Intercept, and Punch *Chin Pu Pan Lan Chui*

Movement 1: Move your right fist in an arc back to the right side of your waist. Begin to bring your left hand up. At the same time, slowly shift your weight to your right foot, and take one big step forward with your left foot. Push your left arm forward, your palm facing downward, your fingertips pointing upward, and your elbow slightly bent. (See photo 72A.)

Eyes: Follow your left hand.
Breathing: Inhale.
Mind: Concentrate on the dantian.
Self-Defense: Use your left arm and hand to protect your chest.

Movement 2: Shift your weight to your left foot, bending the knee, and punch your right fist forward at chest height. The bottom of your fist should face inward. At the same time, pull your left hand back next to your right forearm, near the elbow. (See photo 72B.)

Eyes: Follow both arms and hands.
Breathing: Exhale.
Mind: Visualize energy coming from the dantian through both arms to both hands, then to your right fist and left palm.
Self-Defense: Use your right fist to attack an opponent in front of you and your left arm and hand to protect your chest.

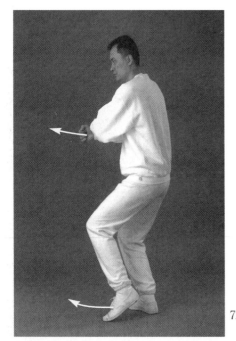

72A

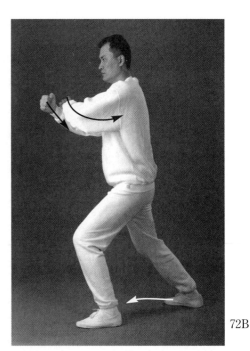

72B

(73) Step Forward and Ward Off, Right *Shang Pu Yu Peng*

Movement 1: Shift the all weight to the left foot, and put your left hand at the height of your throat with your palm down and elbow bent. Move your right hand near the right side of your waist with the palm upward. This posture resembles holding a ball in your hands on the left side of your body. (See photo 73A.)

Eyes: Follow your left hand.
Breathing: Inhale.
Mind: Concentrate on the dantian.
Self-Defense: Put more chi on both hands and palms.

Movement 2: Gradually turn the trunk about 45 degrees to the right so that the right foot rises on tiptoe. Touching first with the heel, place the right foot directly to the right side, and slowly shift the weight onto it while turning the upper torso to the right. At the same time, raise the right arm with the elbow slightly down. Continue to raise the right arm until the palm faces your chest; then press your left palm on your right wrist. (See photo 73B.)

Eyes: Follow right upper arm, forearm, and hand.
Breathing: Exhale.
Mind: Direct energy from the dantian to your right arm and hand.
Self-Defense: Use your right upper arm, forearm, and hand to protect yourself against an opponent's attack on your right side.

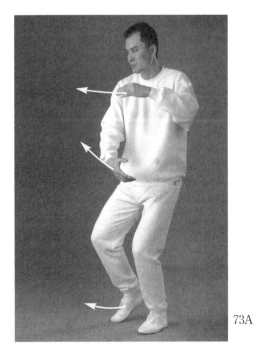

73A

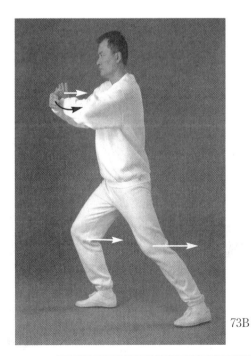

73B

(74) Withdraw and Push *Ju Feng Shih Pi*

Movement 1: Turn both palms down as the left hand passes over the right wrist and moves forward and then left, ending level with the right hand. Separate hands a shoulder's width apart, and "sit" back as you shift your weight to the slightly bent right leg. Draw both hands back to the front of the abdomen, palms facing slightly downward to the front. (See photo 74A.)

Eyes: Look forward.
Breathing: Inhale.
Mind: Concentrate on the dantian.
Self-Defense: Use both arms and hands to grasp your opponent's shoulders toward you and pull down.

Movement 2: Slowly transfer your weight to the left leg while pushing your hands forward and obliquely up, palms facing forward, until your wrists are shoulder high. At the same time, bend the left knee into a bow step. (See photo 74B.)

Eyes: Follow both hands.
Breathing: Exhale.
Mind: Visualize energy coming from the dantian through both arms to both hands.
Self-Defense: Use both hands to push your opponent's chest away.

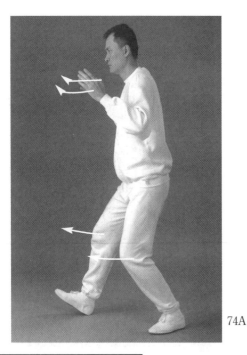

74A

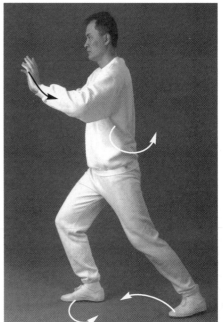

74B

(75) Single Whip *Tan Pien*

Movement 1: Shift your weight gradually to the left foot. Turn your torso to the left 180 degrees and, at the same time, swivel on the right heel, curving the toes inward as far as possible. As you shift your weight back to the right leg, allow the body to turn to the right and, as the elbow bends, withdraw the right arm. Allow the fingers to point downward and close them at the fingertips, forming a "hook" near the right armpit. Bring the left hand to rest, palm up, near the right breast. (See photo 75A.)

Eyes: Follow your right hand.
Breathing: Inhale.
Mind: Concentrate on the dantian.
Self-Defense: Use your right hand to protect yourself when an opponent closes in on your right side.

Movement 2: As the torso turns toward the left, take a wide step to the left with the left foot. First set the heel down, then the toes, which point left. Shift your weight to the left leg. The left heel should not be directly in front of the right heel but on as wide a diagonal position as you can comfortably manage. Gradually shift the body weight to your left leg, bending the leg at the knee. At the same time, turn the left palm outward with arm slightly bent. (See photo 75B.)

Eyes: Follow your left hand.
Breathing: Exhale.
Mind: Visualize energy coming from the dantian through your left arm to your left hand.
Self-Defense: Use your left hand to attack an opponent on your left side.

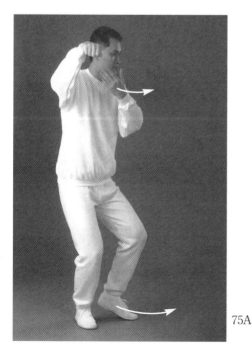

75A

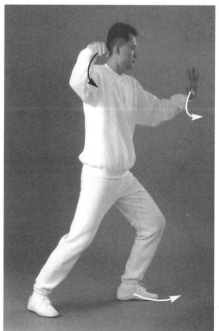

75B

Movement 1: Shift your weight to your right foot. Slowly bend your right knee and extend the left foot to your side, slightly touching the floor. At the same time, let your left hand fall down in an arc across the inside of your left leg. Slowly lower your body as far as your right knee can bend. Do not force yourself; your flexibility will improve over time. Finish the arc with your left hand by bringing it above your outstretched leg, and start to bring the hand up. Keep your right hand in the "hook" and start to bring it, in an arc, down to your hip. (See photo 76A.)

Eyes: Follow your left hand.
Breathing: Inhale.
Mind: Visualize energy coming from the dantian through your left arm to your left hand.
Self-Defense: Use your left arm and hand to protect your lower body.

Movement 2: Turn your left toes outward as far as possible. Use your heel as the axis. Shift your weight to the left foot, and bend your left knee. Extend your right leg and turn your toes inward. Slightly turn your upper body to the left. Raise yourself up with a forward movement as you shift your weight. At the same time, move your right hand in an arc forward and up to shoulder level, crossing with the left hand in front of your chest. (See photo 76B.)

Eyes: Follow your right hand.
Breathing: Exhale.
Mind: Visualize energy coming from the dantian through your right arm to your right hand.
Self-Defense: Use the right arm and hand to protect yourself against an attack in front of you.

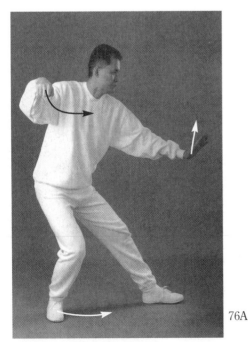

76A

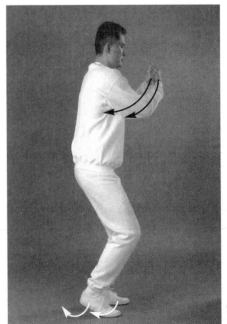

76B

(77) Turn Around and Strike with Right Foot *Ch'uan Shen Teng Cho*

Movement 1: Put your right foot down a half step next to your left foot. Draw both hands near to the body and cross them in front of your chest. Raise your left leg with knee bent and foot suspended in the air next to your right leg. Then swing your body to the right about 360 degrees by turning on your right heel. Put your left foot down a half step next to your right foot. Shift your weight to your left foot. (See photo 77A.)

Eyes: Look forward.
Breathing: Inhale.
Mind: Concentrate on the dantian.
Self-Defense: Put more chi on both hands and the right foot.

Movement 2: Kick forward with the sole of your right foot with toes upward, while chopping forward with both hands at the level of your chest. (See photo 77B.)

Eyes: Follow both hands and the right foot.
Breathing: Exhale.
Mind: Visualize energy coming from the dantian through both arms to both hands and through the right leg to the right foot.
Self-Defense: Use both arms and hands as well as your right foot to attack an opponent in front of you.

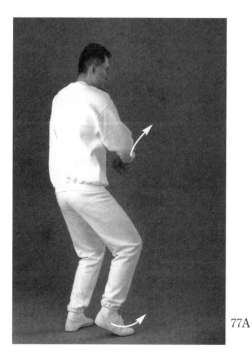

77A

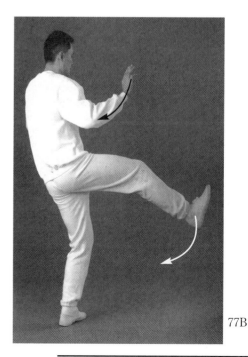

77B

(78) Chop with Fist *Pieh Shen Chui*

Movement 1: Pull your right foot next to your left. At the same time, make a fist with your right hand, and move it past the left rib cage with the fist pointing down. Your left palm should face forward. (See photo 78A.)

Eyes: Look forward.
Breathing: Inhale.
Mind: Concentrate on the dantian.
Self-Defense: Put more chi on both hands and the right fist.

Movement 2: Take one big step forward with your right foot, letting the heel touch the floor first. Slowly shift your weight to your right foot. Snap your fist forward and out, fully extending the arm. (See photo 78B.)

Eyes: Follow your right fist.
Breathing: Exhale.
Mind: Visualize chi coming from the dantian through your right arm to your right fist.
Self-Defense: Use your right fist to attack an opponent in front of you.

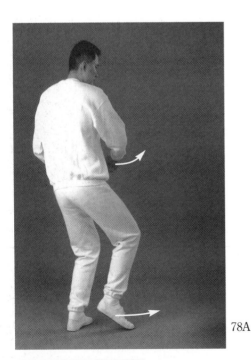

78A

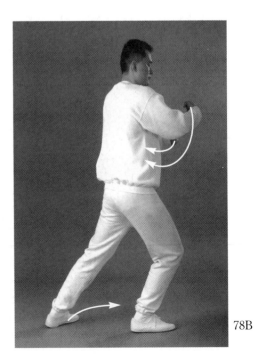

78B

(79) Step, Deflect, Intercept, and Punch *Chin Pu Pan Lan Chui*

Movement 1: Move your right fist, in an arc, back to the right side of your waist. Begin to bring your left hand up. At the same time, slowly shift your weight to your right foot and take one big step forward with your left foot. Push your left arm forward, the palm facing downward and your fingertips pointing upward, with elbow slightly bent. (See photo 79A.)

Eyes: Follow your left hand.
Breathing: Inhale.
Mind: Concentrate on the dantian.
Self-Defense: Use your left arm and hand to protect your chest.

Movement 2: Shift your weight to your left foot, bending the knee, and punch your right fist forward at chest height. The bottom of your fist should face inward. At the same time, pull your left hand back next to your right forearm, near the elbow. (See photo 79B.)

Eyes: Follow both arms and hands.
Breathing: Exhale.
Mind: Visualize energy coming from the dantian through both arms to both hands, then to the right fist and left palm.
Self-Defense: Use your right fist to attack an opponent in front of you and your left arm and hand to protect your chest.

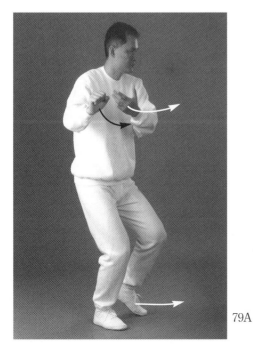

79A

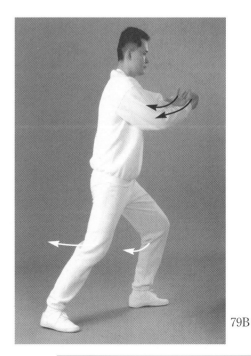

79B

(80) Withdraw and Push *Ju Feng Shih Pi*

Movement 1: Turn both palms down as the left hand passes over the right wrist and moves forward and then left, ending level with the right hand. Separate hands a shoulder's width apart, and "sit" back as you shift your weight to the slightly bent right leg. Draw both hands back to the front of the abdomen, palms facing slightly downward to the front. (See photo 80A.)

Eyes: Look forward.
Breathing: Inhale.
Mind: Concentrate on the dantian.
Self-Defense: Use both arms and hands to grasp your opponent's shoulders toward you and pull down.

Movement 2: Slowly transfer your weight to the left leg while pushing your hands forward and obliquely up, palms facing forward, until your wrists are shoulder high. At the same time, bend the left knee into a bow step. (See photo 80B.)

Eyes: Follow both hands.
Breathing: Exhale.
Mind: Visualize energy coming from the dantian through both arms to both hands.
Self-Defense: Use both hands to push your opponent's chest away.

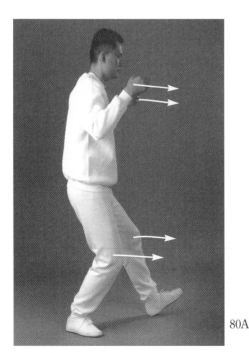

80A

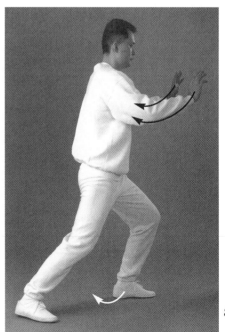

80B

(81) Crossing Hands *Shih Tsu Shou*

Movement: Shift your weight to the right leg, and turn your body to the right with your left heel touching the ground. Bend your right knee and "sit" back (see photo). Following the turn of the body, move both hands to your sides in a circular movement at shoulder level, palms facing forward and elbows slightly bent. Slowly shift your weight to the left leg, and turn the toes of your right foot inward. Then bring your right foot toward the left so that both feet are parallel and a shoulder's width apart. Gradually straighten the legs. At the same time, move both hands down and cross them in front of your abdomen. Raise crossed hands to chest level with your wrists at shoulder level, your right hand on the outside, and your palms facing inward. (See photo 81.)

Eyes: Look forward.
Breathing: Inhale.
Mind: Concentrate on the dantian.
Self-Defense: Use both arms and hands to protect your chest.

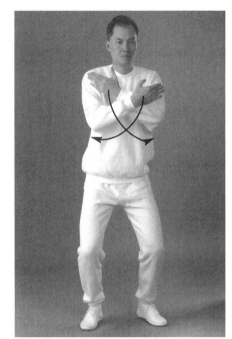

81

(82) Closing *Shou Shi*

Movement: Turn palms forward and downward while lowering both hands gradually to the side of your hips. (See photo 82.)

Eyes: Look forward.
Breathing: Exhale.
Mind: Visualize energy coming from the dantian through both legs to your feet.
Self-Defense: Strengthen both legs and feet by moving the energy down.

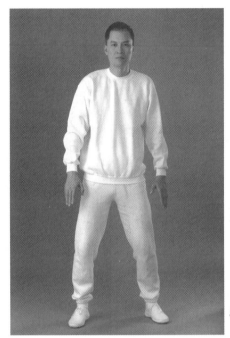

82

A Quick Review of New-Style Tai Chi Ch'uan Forms
First Sequence (Forms 1–20)

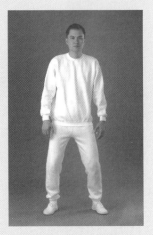

(1) *Yu Pei Shih*
Preparation

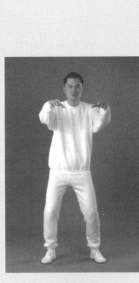

(2) *Chi Shin*
Beginning

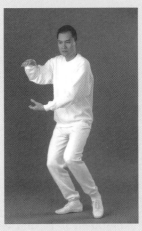

(3) *Tso Peng*
Ward Off, Left

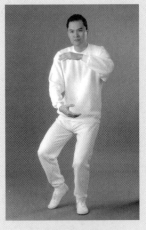

(4) *Yu Peng*
Ward Off, Right

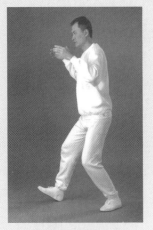

(5) *Ju Feng Shih Pi*
Withdraw and Push

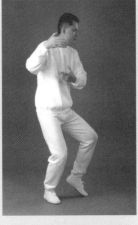

(7) *Tso Lou Shi Yao Pu*
Brush Left Knee and
Twist Step

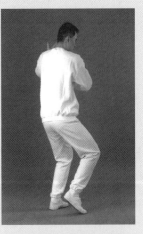

(8) *Yu Lou Shi Yao Pu*
Brush Right Knee and
Twist Step

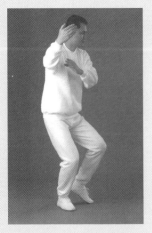

(9) *Tso Lou Shi Yao Pu*
Brush Left Knee and
Twist Step

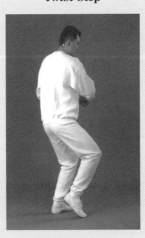

(6) *Tan Pien*
Single Whip

(10) *Pieh Shen Chui*
Chop with Fist

First Sequence (Forms 1–20)

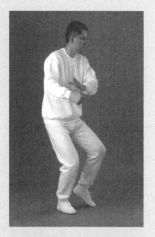

(11) *Chin Pu Pan Lan Chui*
Step, Deflect, Intercept,
and Punch

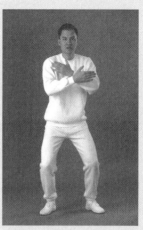

(13) Shih Tsu Shou
Crossing Hands

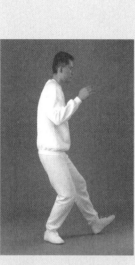

(12) *Ju Feng Shih Pi*
Withdraw and Push

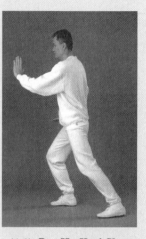

(14) *Pao Hu Kuei Shan*
Embrace the Tiger and
Return to the Mountain

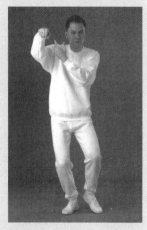

(15) *Hsieh Tan Pien*
Slanting Single Whip

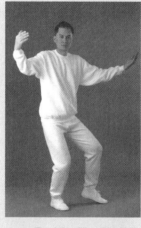

(17) *Tao Nien Hou, Yu Shih*
Step Back and Drive
the Monkey Away, Right

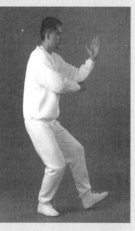

(16) *Chou Ti Chui*
Punch under Elbow

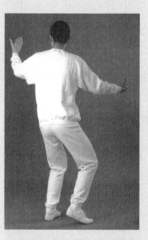

(18) *Tao Nien Hou, Tso Shih*
Step Back and Drive
the Monkey Away, Left

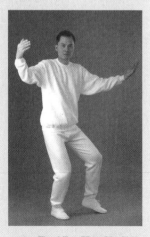

(19) *Tao Nien Hou, Yu Shih*
Step Back and Drive
the Monkey Away, Right

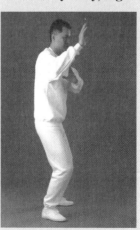

(20) *Hsieh Fei Shih*
Diagonal Flying
Posture

Second Sequence (Forms 21–40)

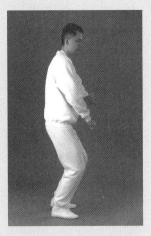

(21) *Kao*
Shoulder Stroke

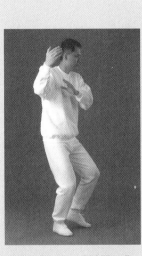

(22) *Tso Lou Shi Yao Pu*
Brush Left Knee and
Twist Step

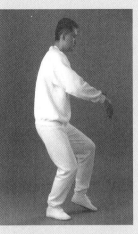

(23) *Hai Ti Chen*
Needle at the Bottom
of the Sea

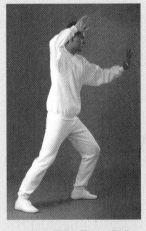

(24) *Shan Tjung Pei*
Fan Penetrates the
Back

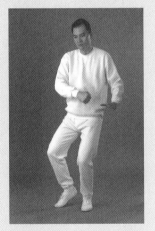

(25) *Ch'uan Shen Pieh
Shen Chui*
Turn Around and Chop

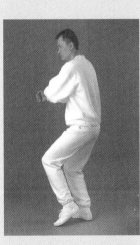

(26) *Chin Pu Pan Lan Chui*
Step, Deflect,
Intercept, and Punch

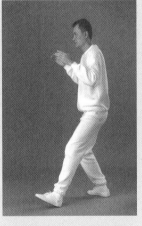

(27) *Ju Feng Shih Pi*
Withdraw and Push

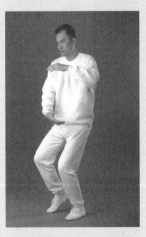

(28) *Shang Pu Yu Peng*
Step Forward and
Ward Off, Right

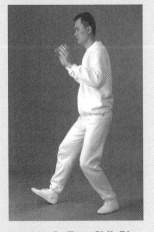

(29) *Ju Feng Shih Pi*
Withdraw and Push

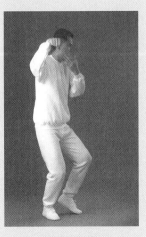

(30) *Tan Pien*
Single Whip

Second Sequence (Forms 21–40)

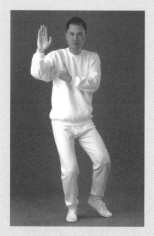

(31) *Yun Shou*
Waving Hands in
Clouds

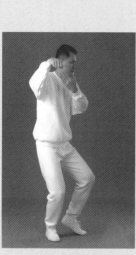

(32) *Tan Pien*
Single Whip

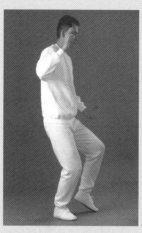

(33) *Kao Tan Ma*
High Pat on Horse

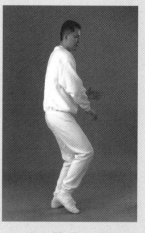

(34) *Yu Teng Cho*
Strike with Right Foot

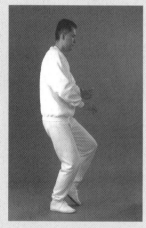

(35) *Tso Teng Cho*
Strike with Left Foot

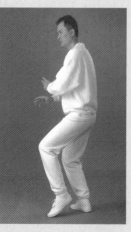

(36) *Ch'uan Shen Teng Cho*
Turn Around and
Strike with Left Foot

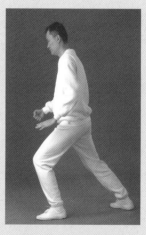

(37) *Chin Pu Tsai Chui*
Step Forward and
Punch Downward

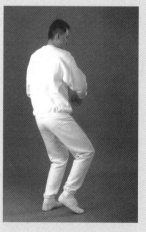

(38) *Ch'uan Shen Pieh Shien Chui*
Turn Around and Chop
with Fist

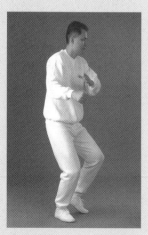

(39) *Chin Pu Pan Lan Chui*
Step, Deflect,
Intercept, and Punch

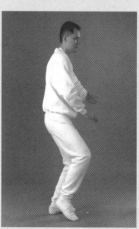

(40) *Yu Teng Cho*
Strike with Right Foot

Third Sequence (Forms 41–60)

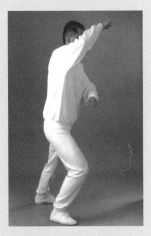

(41) *Ta Hu Shih*
Strike the Tiger

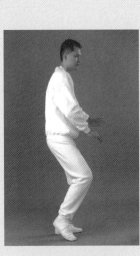

(42) *Yu Teng Cho*
Strike with Right Foot

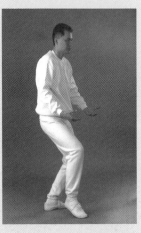

(43) *Shuang Feng Kuan Er*
Strike with Both Fists

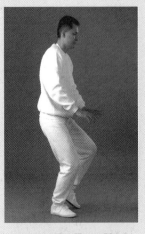

(44) *Tso Teng Cho*
Strike with Left Foot

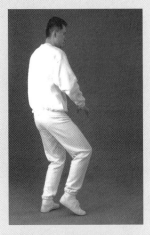

(45) *Ch'uan Shen Teng Cho*
Turn Around and
Strike with Right Foot

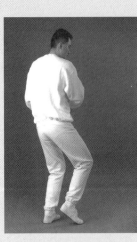

(46) *Pieh Shen Chui*
Chop with Fist

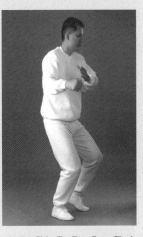

(47) *Chin Pu Pan Lan Chui*
Step, Deflect,
Intercept, and Punch

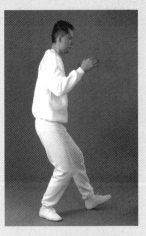

(48) *Ju Feng Shih Pi*
Withdraw and Push

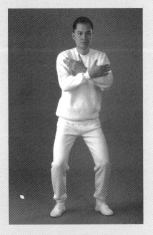

(49) *Shih Tsu Shou*
Crossing Hands

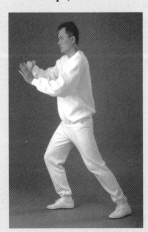

(50) *Yu Peng*
Ward Off, Right

Third Sequence (Forms 41–60)

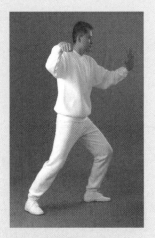

(51) *Tan Pien*
Single Whip

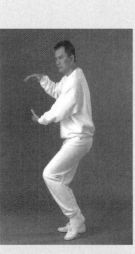

(52) *Yu Nu Ch'uan Sho*
**Fair Lady Weaving at
the Shuttle I**

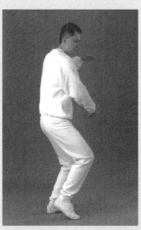

(53) *Yu Nu Ch'uan Sho*
**Fair Lady Weaving at
the Shuttle II**

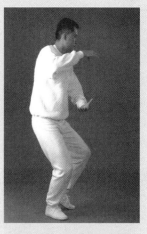

(54) *Yu Nu Ch'uan Sho*
**Fair Lady Weaving at
the Shuttle III**

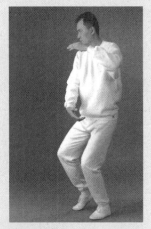

(55) *Yu Nu Ch'uan Sho*
**Fair Lady Weaving at
the Shuttle IV**

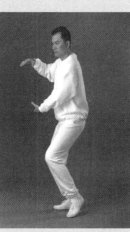

(56) *Tso Peng*
Ward Off, Left

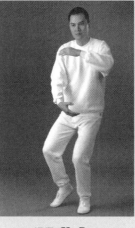

(57) *Yu Peng*
Ward Off, Right

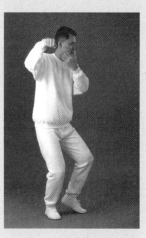

(58) *Tan Pien*
Single Whip

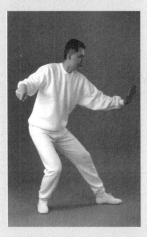

(59) *Tan Pien Hsia Shih*
**Single Whip Squatting
Down**

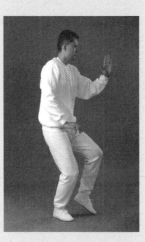

(60) *Tso Lou Hsih Yao Pu*
**Brush Left Knee and
Twist Step**

Fourth Sequence (Forms 61–82)

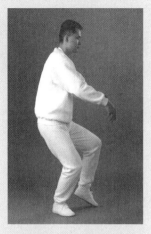

(61) *Hai Ti Chen*
Needle at the Bottom
of the Sea

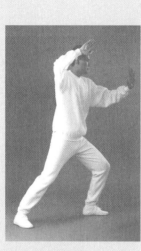

(62) *Shan Tjung Pei*
Fan Penetrates the
Back

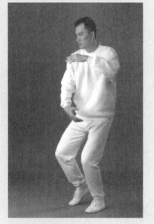

(65) *Shang Pu Yu Peng*
Step Forward and
Ward Off, Right

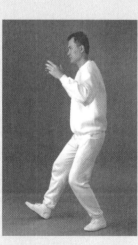

(66) *Ju Feng Shih Pi*
Withdraw and Push

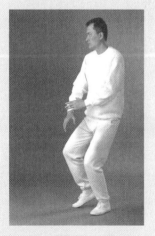

(69) *Yu Teng Cho*
Turn Around and
Strike with Right Foot

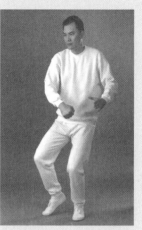

(63) *Ch'uan Shen Pieh
Shen Chui*
Turn Around and Chop

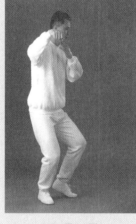

(67) *Tan Pien*
Single Whip

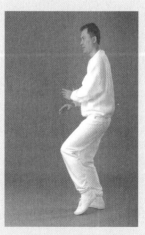

(70) *Tso Teng Cho*
Strike with Left Foot

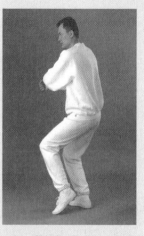

(64) *Chin Pu Pan Lan Chui*
Step, Deflect,
Intercept, and Punch

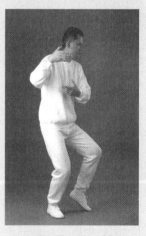

(68) *Kao Tan Ma*
High Pat on Horse

Fourth Sequence (Forms 61–82)

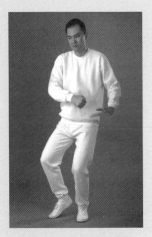

(71) *Chin Pu Tsai Chui*
Step Forward and
Punch Downward

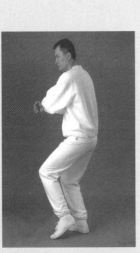

(72) *Chin Pu Pan Lan Chui*
Step, Deflect,
Intercept, and Punch

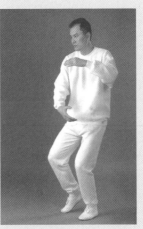

(73) *Shang Pu Yu Peng*
Step Forward and
Ward Off, Right

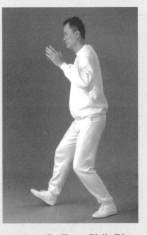

(74) *Ju Feng Shih Pi*
Withdraw and Push

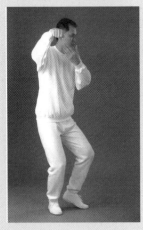

(75) *Tan Pien*
Single Whip

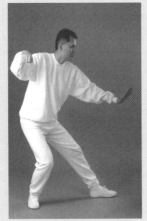

(76) *Tan Pien Hsia Shih*
Single Whip Squatting
Down

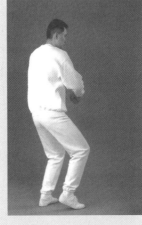

(77) *Ch'uan Shen Teng Cho*
Turn Around and
Strike with Right Foot

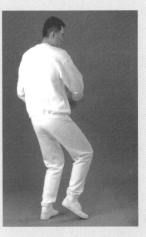

(78) *Pieh Shen Chui*
Chop with Fist

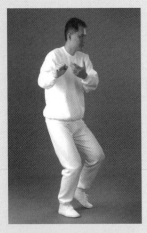

(79) *Chin Pu Pan Lan Chui*
Step, Deflect, Intercept,
and Punch

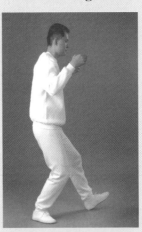

(80) *Ju Feng Shih Pi*
Withdraw and Push

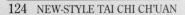

Fourth Sequence (Forms 61–82)

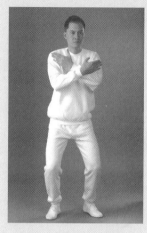

(81) *Shih Tsu Shou*
Crossing Hands

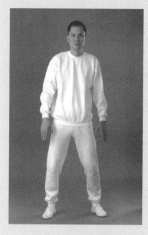

(82) Shou *Shi*
Closing

These photos illustrate the first movement of each of the 82 forms of New-Style Tai Chi Ch'uan.

About the Authors

Wei Yue Sun graduated with a medical degree in 1988 from the Sun Yat-Sen University of Medical Sciences in Guangzhou, People's Republic of China. He is a U.S. Medical License Exam / Education Commission for Foreign Medical Graduates board-certified medical doctor and currently a resident in internal medicine at Brookdale University Hospital and Medical Center in Brooklyn, New York. He had been a clinical and public health epidemiologist in the New York City Department of Health. Dr. Sun has practiced both traditional Chinese medicine and Western medicine in China and in the United States. As a tai chi ch'uan master, he has taught different styles of tai chi ch'uan for many years in both countries.

Xiao Jing Li graduated from Guangzhou Medical College in Guangzhou, People's Republic of China, in 1986. She is a U.S. National Certification Commission for Acupuncture & Oriental Medicine board-certified medical doctor and has practiced traditional Chinese medicine and Western medicine for over 10 years. She is a research associate in molecular biology at City University of New York. Dr. Li has practiced and taught tai chi ch'uan as well as acupuncture and Chinese herbal medicine for many years in both China and the United States, most recently in her natural healing center in Brooklyn, New York. She has also developed new therapies that combine ancient Chinese medical theories and modern Western medical techniques.

Dr. Sun and Dr. Li, husband and wife, have done research in tai chi ch'uan and its effects on health and well-being. The tai chi ch'uan techniques presented in this book are the result of years of practice and scientific research.

Dr. Sun and Dr. Li coauthored the book *Chi Kung: Increase Your Energy, Improve Your Health* (Sterling, 1997). With William Chen, Ph.D., Dr. Sun coauthored another tai-chi book, *Tai Chi Ch'uan: The Gentle Workout for Mind & Body* (Sterling, 1995).

Index

A

acupuncture/acupressure, 15, 19, 20, 26;
    see also channels (eight); meridians
    (twelve)
  as anesthetic, 19
  German neo-, 20
  points, 17, 19–20
  tobiscope and, 19
  types, 17, 20
Anhui province, 10
arrows, use on photos, 35
attacking/being attacked, 9–10, 24, 30–31

B

Beginning (Form 2), 34, 36, 117
Beijing Short-Form Tai Chi Ch'uan, 10
Belt Channel, 15, 16
bioelectrography, 20
Bladder Meridian, 17–18
body and mind, 14, 21–22
body processes and cosmos, 8
breathing, 7, 10–11, 13, 21
  abdominal, 7, 23–24
  body as dirty leather bag, 23
  from dantian and heels, 7–8
  fetal, 23–24
  oxygen and elements, 23
  prenatal and postnatal, 7, 23–24
  with throat, 7, 23
Brush Left Knee and Twist Step (Forms
  7, 9, 22, 60), 34, 41, 42, 56, 94, 119,
  122
Buddhism, 9, 10, 21, 23

C

Chang San-Feng, 9
channels (eight), 8, 15–17, 19, 21–22
  belt (*Tai Mo*), 15, 16
  control (*Tu Mo*), 15, 16
  function (*Jen Mo*), 15, 16
  negative arm (*Yin Yu Wei Mo*), 15, 16
  negative leg (*Yin Chiao Mo*), 15, 16, 17
  positive arm (*Yang Yu Wei Mo*), 15, 16
  positive leg (*Yang Chiao Mo*), 15, 16
  thrusting (*Cheung Mo*), 15, 16
Cheung Mo (Thrusting Channel), 15, 16
chi (vital energy), 8, 10, 13, 15, 19, 20,
  21–22, 26; *see also* breathing; meditation
  becomes spirit, 28
  bow and arrow metaphor, 24
  circulation, 7–8, 15, 23

chi (vital energy) (*cont.*)
  dantian, originating in, 8
  detecting, 19–20
  flowing through channels and meridi-
    ans, 15–20, 21–22, 23–24, 26
  meditation and, 21–22
  tai chi ch'uan aiding, 26
  wind metaphor, 24
chi kung, 10, 15
Chinese medicine, traditional, 12–14, 15,
  19–20, 22, 26, 27–29
Chinese National Physical Education
  Association (CNPEA), 10–11
Chinese philosophies
  Buddhism, 9, 10, 21
  Confucianism, 9, 21, 23
  Taoism, 9, 10, 12, 13, 21, 23–24, 28
Chin Pu Pan Lan Chui (Forms 11, 26, 39,
  47, 48, 64, 72, 79), 34, 45, 60, 73, 81,
  98, 106, 113, 118, 119, 120, 121,
  123, 124
Chin Pu Tsai Chui (Forms 37, 71), 34, 71,
  105, 124
Chi Shin (Form 2), 34, 36, 117
Chop with Fist (Forms 10, 46, 78), 34, 44,
  80, 112, 117, 121, 124
Chou Ti Chui (Form 16), 34, 50, 118
Ch'uan Shen Pieh Shen Chui (Forms 25,
  38, 63), 34, 59, 72, 97, 120, 123
Ch'uan Shen Teng Cho (Forms 36, 45,
  77), 34, 70, 79, 111, 120
Chuang Tzu, 7, 8
Closing (Form 82), 34, 116
computer tomography (CT) scan, 20
Confucianism, 9, 21, 23
concentration; *see* meditation
contemplation and turbulence, 7
Control Channel, 15, 16
corn, tale of growing, 34
counterattacking, 30
creativity, 12, 13
Crossing Hands (Forms 13, 39, 49, 81),
  34, 47, 83, 115, 118, 120, 121, 125

D

dantian, 7, 23–24; *and passim*
  defined, 7
Diagonal Flying Posture (Form 20), 34,
  54, 118
disease, prevention or cure, 8, 27–28
dualism, 12; *see* yin and yang

E

eight channels, 15–17
elements in the air, 23
Embrace the Tiger and Return to the
  Mountain (Form 14), 34, 48, 118
energy, vital; *see* chi
eye movements, 10, 11
exercise
  age and tai chi ch'uan, 25
  breathing coordinated, 23–24
  fitness and regular, 25–26
  gentle, 25
  leg muscles and, 25–26
  with meditation, 8, 9, 10, 25, 26
  Shao Lin method of, 9
  sex and, 12–13
  stress-reduction, 26
  variety, 26
  walled city metaphor, 8
  yin and yang, 12–14, 23–24

F

Fair Lady Weaving at Shuttle I–IV
  (Forms 52–55), 22, 34, 86–89
Fan Penetrates the Back (Forms 24, 62),
  34, 58, 96, 119, 122, 123
farmer from village of Sung, 24
First Sequence (Forms 1–20), 34, 35–54,
  117–118
forms (eighty-two) New-Style Tai Chi
  Ch'uan; *see also specific forms*
  with instructions and photos, 35–116
  list , 34
  quick review (photos), 117–125
Fourth Sequence (Forms 61–82), 34,
  95–116, 124–125
Function Channel, 15, 16

G

Gaikin, Dr. Mikhail Kuzmich, 19
Gallbladder Meridian, 17–18
Great Quiescence, 24

H

Hai Ti Chen (Forms 23, 61), 34, 57, 95
health benefits of tai chi ch'uan, 27–29
  disease, protection from, 27
  heart, 27–28
  kidneys, 28
  liver, 28
  lungs, 27
  mental and emotional, 27, 28–29
    anger, 29

health benefits of tai chi ch'uan (*cont.*)
  mental and emotional
    desire, 29
    fear, 29
    grief, 28
    tension, 26, 29
  muscles, 25–26, 28
  relaxation, 26
  skeleton, 28
  stress-reduction, 26, 29
Heart Governor Meridian, 18–19
Heart Meridian, 17–18
heels, breathing from, 7–8
High Pat on Horse (Forms 33, 68), 34, 67, 102, 123
holy fetus, 7
Hsieh Fei Shih (Form 20), 34, 54, 118
Hsieh Tan Pien (Form 15), 34, 49, 118
Huai Chin Nan, 10
Huang Ti, 12
Hua To, 8–9

I

I Ching (*Book of Changes*), 7, 8, 10, 12
illness, preventing and curing, 27–28
immortality, 13
Inner School (Shao Lin method) v. Outer School (tai chi ch'uan), 9

J

Japanese shiatsu, 20
Jen Mo (Function Channel), 15, 16
Ju Feng Shih Pi (Forms 5, 12, 27, 29, 40, 46, 48, 66, 74, 80), 34, 39, 61, 82, 100, 108, 114, 117, 118, 119, 121, 123, 124

K

Kao (Form 21), 34, 55, 119
Kao Tan Ma (Forms 33, 68), 34, 67, 102, 120, 123
Kidney Meridian, 17–18
Kirlian, Semyon Davidovich, 19
  photography (bioelectrography), 19–20
knee injuries and tai chi ch'uan, 25–26
Ko Hung, 9

L

Lao Tzu, 7
Large Intestine Meridian, 17–18
leg work (muscles), 25–26, 28
Liver Meridian, 18–19
longevity, 12, 13, 14, 24
Lu Kuan Yu, 10
Lung Meridian, 17–18

M

magnetic resonance imaging (MRI), 20
martial arts (self-defense), 9–10, 30–31
meditation, 23–24
  breathing and, 23–24

meditation (*cont.*)
  goal of, 24
  moving, 21
  sitting, 21
  with tai chi ch'uan, 13–14, 22
meridians (twelve), 15, 17–19, 21–22
  bladder, 17, 18
  centrifugal/centripetal, 17, 19
  detecting, 19–20
  fixed direction of, 17
  gallbladder, 17, 18
  heart, 17, 18
  heart governor, 17, 18, 19
  kidney, 17, 18
  large intestine, 17, 18
  liver, 17, 18, 19
  small intestine, 17, 18, 19
  spleen, 17, 18
  stomach, 17, 18
  triple warmer, 17, 18
  yin and yang designation of, 17
Mikalevsky, Vladislov, 19
movement(s)
  animal, 8–9
  arrows on photos, 35
  eye, 10–11
  and meditation, 13–14, 21–22
  with stillness, 8
Movement of the Five Animals, 8–9
moving meditation, 21
muscle memory, 10
muscle work, 9–10, 25–26, 28

N

Needle at the Bottom of the Sea (Forms 23, 61), 34, 35, 57, 85, 119, 123
Negative Arm Channel, 16
Negative Leg Channel, 16–17
neo-acupuncture, German, 20
New-Style Tai Chi Ch'uan Forms, 33–125
  arrows, direction of movement and, 35
  First Sequence (Forms 1–20), 34, 35–54, 117–118
  forms (82) with instructions and photos, 35–116
  Fourth Sequence (Forms 61–82), 34, 95–116, 124–125
  list of 82 forms, 34
  quick review of, 117–125
  Second Sequence (Forms 21–40), 34, 55–74, 119–120
  Third Sequence (Forms 41–60), 34, 75–94, 121–122
New-Style Tai Chi Ch'uan, history, 10–11
  CNPEA and, 10–11
Nixon, Richard (former U.S. President), 19

O

official Chinese system (1993), 11
Outer School (tai chi ch'uan) v. Inner School (Shao Lin method), 9

P

Pao Hu Kuei Shan (Form 14), 34, 48, 118
physical immortality, 13, 23
physiological foundation, 15
Pieh Shen Chui (Forms 10, 46, 47, 78), 34, 44, 80, 112, 117, 121, 124
People's Republic of China, 10–11
  CNPEA, 10–11
  physical education classes, 11
points, acupuncture/ acupressure, 19–20
  as anesthetic, 19
  sedation, 17
  source, 17
  tonification, 17
positron emission tomography (PET) scan, 20
Positive Arm Channel, 15, 16
Positive Leg Channel, 15, 16
Preparation (Form 1), 6, 7–8, 34, 35, 117
Punch under Elbow (Form 16), 34, 50, 118

Q

A Quick Review of New-Style Tai Chi Forms, 117–125

R

relaxation, 21, 26
rest (yin) and movement (yang), 12; *see also* yin and yang

S

scientific investigation of channels and meridians, 15, 19–20
Second Sequence (Forms 21–40), 34, 55–74, 119–120
Secrets of Chinese Meditation (book), 10
sedation points, 17
self-defense skills, 7, 9–10, 30–31
sexual energy, 12–13
Shang Pu Yu Peng (Forms 28, 65, 73), 34, 62, 99, 107, 119, 123, 124
Shan Tjung Pei (Forms 24, 62), 34, 58, 96, 119, 123
Shao Lin method, 9–10
shiatsu, 20
Shih Tsu Shou (Forms 13, 49, 81), 34, 47, 83, 115, 118, 121, 125
Shoulder Stroke (Form 21), 34, 55, 119
Shou Shi (Form 82), 34, 116, 125
Shuang Feng Kuan Er (Form 43), 34, 77, 121
Single Whip (Forms 6, 30, 32, 51, 58, 67, 75), 34, 40, 64, 66, 85, 92, 101, 109,

Single Whip (*cont.*)
117, 119, 120, 122, 123, 124
Single Whip Squatting Down (Forms 59, 76), 34, 93, 110, 124
sitting meditation, 21
Slanting Single Whip (Form 15), 34, 49, 118
Small Intestine Meridian, 18–19
source points, 17
Spleen Meridian, 17–18
Step, Deflect, Intercept, and Punch (Forms 11, 26, 39, 47, 64, 72, 73, 79, 81), 34, 45, 60, 73, 81, 98, 100, 113, 117, 119, 120, 121, 123, 124, 125
Step Back and Drive the Monkey Away (*Tao Nien Hu*), 8
Left (Form 18), 34, 52, 118
Right (Forms 17, 19), 34, 51, 118
Step Forward and Punch Downward (Forms 37, 71), 34, 71, 105, 120, 124
Step Forward and Ward Off, Right (Forms 28, 65, 73), 34, 35, 62, 99, 107, 119, 123, 124
Stomach Meridian, 17–18
stress-reduction, 26, 29
Strike the Tiger (Form 41), 34, 75, 121
Strike with Both Fists (Form 43), 34, 77, 123
Strike with Left Foot (Forms 35, 44, 70), 34, 69, 78, 104, 120, 121, 123
Strike with Right Foot (Forms 34, 40, 42, 45), 34, 68, 74, 76, 120, 121, 123
suffering and emotions, 28–29
Sung village and corn farmer, 34
supreme ultimate (*Tai Chi Tu*), 13
surgery, acupuncture as anesthetic, 19

T

Ta Hu Shih (Form 41), 34, 75, 121
Tai Chi Tu diagram (Supreme Ultimate), 13
tai chi ch'uan, 10, 15
age and practice, 25
Beijing Short Form, 10
breathing and (exercise of yin and yang), 23–24
and fitness, 25
forms, 34, 35–116, 117–125
as gentle exercise, 25
health benefits, 13, 27–29
history, 7–11
knee injuries with, 25–26
meditation and flow of chi, 21–22
as moving meditation, 21–22
New Style, 10–11, 33–125
philosophy (yin and yang), 12–14
physical movements, 25–26, 35–116

tai chi ch'uan (*cont.*)
physiology (channels and meridians), 12–14
as self-defense, 30–31
stress-reduction, 26, 29
understanding, 5–32
Tai Mo (Belt Channel), 15, 16
Ta Mo, master, 9
Tan Pien (Forms 6, 30, 32, 51, 58, 67, 75), 34, 40, 64, 66, 85, 92, 101, 109, 117, 191, 122, 123, 124
Tan Pien Hsia Shih (Forms 59, 76), 34, 93, 110, 122, 124
Tao Nien Hou, Tso Shih (Form 18), 34, 52, 118
Tao Nien Hou, Yu Shih (Forms 17, 19), 34, 51, 53, 118
Tao Te Ching, 7
Tao Yin, 9
Taoism
breathing and, 23
opposing manifestations, yin and yang, 12–14
philosophy, 9, 10, 12, 13, 21, 23, 28
Third Sequence (Forms 41–60), 34, 75–94, 121–122
Thrusting Channel, 15, 16
tobiscope, 19
tonification points, 17
traditional Chinese medicine, 12–14, 15, 19–20, 22, 26, 27–29
Western interest, 19–20
Triple Warmer Meridian, 17–18
Tsan Tung Chi (book) (*The Kinship of the Three*), 8
Tso Lou Shi Yao Pu (Forms 7, 9, 22, 60), 34, 43, 56, 94, 117, 119, 122
Tso Peng (Forms 3, 56), 34, 37, 90, 117, 122
Tso Teng Cho (Forms 35, 44, 70), 34, 69, 78, 104, 119, 121, 123
Tu Mo (Control Channel), 15, 16
Turn Around and Chop (Forms 25, 63), 34, 35, 59, 97, 119, 120, 123
Turn Around and Chop with Fist (Form 38), 34, 72, 120
Turn Around and Strike with Left Foot (Form 36), 34, 70, 120
Turn Around and Strike with Right Foot (Forms 45, 69, 77), 34, 79, 103, 111, 124
Twelve Meridians, 17–20

U

Understanding Tai Chi Ch'uan, 5–32

V

vital energy; *see* chi

W

Ward Off, Left (Forms 3, 56), 34, 37, 90, 117, 122
Ward Off, Right (Forms 4, 50, 57), 34, 38, 83, 91, 117, 121, 122
Warring States period, 8
Waving Hands in Clouds (Form 31), 34, 65, 120
Wei Po-Yang, 8
Western World
German neo-acupuncture, 20
renewed interest in traditional Chinese medicine, 19–20, 23
science and medicine, 12, 15, 19–20
White Crane Spreads Its Wings (*Bai He Liang Chi*), 8
Withdraw and Push (Forms 5, 12, 27, 29, 44, 48, 63, 66, 74, 80), 34, 39, 46, 61, 63, 82, 100, 108, 114, 117, 118, 123, 124

X

X rays, 20

Y

Yang Chiao Mo (Positive Leg Channel), 15, 16
Yang Chien Hou, 24
Yang Sheng Chu, 8
Yang Yu Wei Mo (Positive Arm Channel), 15, 16
yin and yang, 8
breathing as exercising, 23–24
"fish," 13
greater/ lesser, 13
manifesting Tao, 12
principles, 12–14
traditional diagram (*Tai Chi Tu*), 13
Yin Chiao Mo (Negative Leg Channel), 15, 16, 17
Yin Shih Tzu, 10
experimental meditation, 10
Secrets of Chinese Meditation (book), 10
Yin Yu Wei Mo (Negative Arm Channel), 16
Yu Lou Shi Yao Pu (Form 8), 34, 42, 117
Yun Shou (Form 31), 34, 65, 120
Yu Nu Ch'uan Sho (Forms 52–55), 34, 86–89, 122
Yu Pei Shih (Form 1), 6, 7–8, 34, 35, 117
Yu Peng (Forms 4, 50, 57), 34, 38, 84, 91, 117, 120, 121, 122
Yu Teng Cho (Forms 34, 40, 42, 69), 34, 68, 76, 103, 120, 121, 123
yung ch'uan cavities, 16–17

Z

Zen, 9, 10; *see also* Buddhism
Zhang Ming, 27